Progress in Hepatology, Volume 3
Hepatocellular Carcinoma

Progress in Hepatology, Volume 3
Hepatocellular Carcinoma

Proceedings of the 'Takahashi Memorial Forum', held in Tokyo, Japan, on 2 November 1996

Editors:

Masami Yamanaka
Teikyo University School of Medicine
Tokyo, Japan

Gotardo Toda
Jikei University School of Medicine
Tokyo, Japan

Teruji Tanaka
Jikei University, Daisan Hospital
Tokyo, Japan

Associate Editors:

Mikio Zeniya
Jikei University School of Medicine
Tokyo, Japan

Hajime Takikawa
Teikyo University School of Medicine
Tokyo, Japan

1997

ELSEVIER

Amsterdam – Lausanne – New York – Oxford – Shannon – Singapore – Tokyo

International Congress Series No. 1142
ISBN 0 444 82678 5

This book is printed on acid-free paper.

Published by:
Elsevier Science B.V.
P.O. Box 211
1000 AE Amsterdam
The Netherlands

In order to ensure rapid publication this volume was prepared using a method of electronic text processing known as Optical Character Recognition (OCR). Specific accuracy and consistency of style were handled by the author. Time did not allow for the usual extensive editing process of the Publisher.

Printed in the Netherlands

Preface

This volume of *Progress in Hepatology* contains articles on basic and clinical research on hepatocellular carcinoma (HCC) in Japan, focusing on its prevention and treatment. These were presented in the meeting of the Third Takahashi Memorial Forum held in Tokyo in 1996. This forum started in 1994 in memory of Professor Tadao Takahashi, the founder of the Japan Society of Hepatology.

The number of patients with HCC is now increasing in Japan. In a recent survey conducted by the Japanese Ministry of Public Health and Welfare, HCC became the third most frequent cause of cancer-related death. In other countries in the Far East, the frequency of HCC-related death is more alarming than in Japan. HCC grows in the chronically injured liver, especially in the case of liver cirrhosis (LC), which is the final outcome of almost all chronic liver diseases. The main cause of chronic liver injury varies from one region in the world to another. In the Far Eastern countries including Japan, the persistent infection with HBV and/or HCV is the most important cause of chronic liver injury. Progress in nutritional therapy and treatment of the major complications of LC, esophageal varices, ascites and encephalopathy, dramatically decreased mortality figures due to LC alone in Japan. Instead, HCC arises as the main cause of death in patients with LC in Japan. In this volume, three chapters deal with the epidemiology, pathology and genomic changes of HCC in Japan.

When patients with HCC-related LC were followed for 10 years or longer, HCC grew in more than half of them. It is therefore necessary to develop a device for the prevention of growth of HCC in the cirrhotic liver. In this volume, three chapters address the trials for the prevention of HCC growth in the chronically injured liver by hepatitis viruses. In the early detection of HCC, ultrasonography is superior to computed tomography, magnetic resonance imaging and determination of serum α-fetoprotein. One chapter deals with the progress in ultrasonography study for early detection of HCC. When HCC is detected early, there are several options for treatment. Six chapters address the therapies adopted in Japan. In these chapters, the indications and limits of these therapies are discussed. One chapter deals with gene therapy as future promising therapy for HCC.

We hope that this volume will help the readers know the present status of HCC and its treatment in Japan, where HCC is prevalent and one of the major causes of cancer-related death.

Gotaru Toda
Professor of Medicine
Jikei University School of Medicine

Contents

Progress in Hepatology, Volume 3.
Hepatocellular Carcinoma.
M. Yamanaka, G. Toda and T. Tanaka, editors.

Epidemiology of hepatitis C virus – associated hepatocellular carcinoma

Kendo Kiyosawa
The Second Department of Internal Medicine, Shinshu University School of Medicine, Matsumoto, Japan

Abstract. Hepatitis virus-related hepatocellular carcinoma (HCC) is distributed worldwide. The distribution of HCC depends on hepatitis B virus (HBV) and hepatitis C virus (HCV) spreading in population in each region. HCV-related HCC is more frequent in Japan and South Europe, in the regions with high prevalence of HCV carriers. Studies in Japan have suggested that the occurrence of HCC increased with time in last 3 decades. Currently, 30,000 HCC patients die per year. Recent advances in genomic analysis indicate that HCV genotype 1b has a risk in progression to HCC.

Keywords: blood transfusion, hepatitis C virus, hepatitis B virus, hepatocellular carcinoma, HCV genotype, male/female ratio, viral genotype.

Introduction

Chronic hepatitis C virus (HCV) infection is a significant public health problem worldwide. HCV is currently recognized as one of the major causes of chronic liver disease; evidence indicates that it also plays a leading role in the development of HCC [1]. Seroepidemiologial study has demonstrated a close relationship among HCV infection, cirrhosis and hepatocellular carcinoma (HCC) [2]. However, analysis of the nucleotide sequence of HCV-RNA isolated from neoplastic and nonneoplastic parts of the liver did not reveal significant genomic differences. There is no information about direct evidence of oncogenesis of HCV so far [3,4].

In this chapter, the geographical, chronological and genomical epidemiologies on HCC are discussed.

Geographical epidemiology

It is well known that the incidence of HCC varies considerably with geographic region, perhaps because of differences in the major causative factors and their frequencies. Bosh and Munoz [5] summarized the age-adjusted incidence rate of HCC based on IARC Scientific Publication (Nos. 75 and 88) as shown in Table 1. In Europe, relatively high rates (> 6.1 per 100,000 pear year in male) are

Address for correspondence: Kendo Kiyosawa MD, The Second Department of Internal Medicine, Shinshu University School of Medicine, 3-1-1, Asahi, Matsumoto 390, Japan. Fax: +81-263-32-9412. E-mail: kkiyosa@gipac.shinshu-u.ac.jp

Table 1. Liver cancer registration worldwide.

Register	Age-adjusted incidence rate per 100,000 population per year		Male/female ratio
	Male	Female	
Europe			
Denmark	3.6	2.3	1.56
Finland	4.0	2.3	1.74
France, Calvados	6.3	0.5	12.60
Germany, Hamburg	4.5	1.7	2.65
Ireland	0.1	0.3	0.77
Italy, Parma	8.6	3.3	2.61
Netherlands	1.0	0.5	2.00
Poland, Warsaw	6.6	4.2	1.57
Spain, Navarra	7.9	4.7	1.68
Switzerland, Basel	8.3	1.4	5.93
United Kingdom	1.6	0.8	2.00
Norway	1.8	1.1	1.64
Africa			
Mozambique	112.9	30.8	3.67
South Africa	28.4	6.9	4.12
Senegal, Dakar	25.6	9.0	2.84
Algeria	1.6	1.4	1.14
Asia			
Philippines, Manila	19.9	6.2	3.21
Korea	13.8	3.2	4.31
China, Shanghai	34.4	11.6	2.97
Hong Kong	32.3	7.4	4.38
India, Bombay	4.9	2.5	1.96
Israel	3.4	1.8	1.89
Japan, Osaka	31.9	7.8	4.09
Hiroshima	20.7	6.0	3.45
Nagasaki	25.8	7.9	3.27
Miyagi	11.2	4.0	2.80
Singapore, Chinese	31.6	7.2	4.39
Indian	14.1	2.8	5.04
Oceania			
New Cadedonia, Melanesian	18.7	5.7	3.28
European	7.9	1.1	7.18
Australia, Capitol area	2.4	0.5	4.80
New Zealand, Maori	11.2	4.2	2.67
Non-Maori	2.4	1.1	2.18
Pacific Polynesia Islands	26.4	2.3	11.48
Hawaii, White	4.2	1.3	3.23
Hawaiian	7.3	2.7	2.70
Japanese	6.2	1.5	4.13
Fiji, Fijian	7.8	4.8	1.63
Indian	1.0	0.4	2.50

(Continued)

Table 1. (Continued).

Register	Age-adjusted incidence rate per 100,000 population per year		Male/female ratio
	Male	Female	
South America			
Argentina, Tandil	9.9	5.8	1.71
Jamaica, Kingston	6.1	2.1	2.90
Cuba	4.1	3.4	1.21
Peru, Lima	4.0	2.9	1.38
Brazil, Recife	9.2	8.3	1.11
North America			
Canada, Eskimos	6.9	3.7	1.86
Alberta	1.3	0.5	2.60
USA (San Francisco)			
Chinese	19.1	3.6	5.31
Black	3.9	1.8	2.17
Japanese	3.0	0.4	7.50
White	2.9	1.1	2.64

Bosh FC and Munoz M. Hepatocellular carcinoma in the world: epidemiologic questions. In Tabor E, DiBisceglie AM, Purcell RH (eds) Etiology, Pathology and Treatment of Hepatocellular Carcinoma in North America. Woodlands Portfolio, 1991;35–54.

seen in Switzerland (Basel), Italy, Spain, France and Poland. Low rates (<2.0 per 100,000 in males) are reported from Norway, United Kingdom, The Netherlands and Ireland. In South America, moderately high rates (>6.1 per 100,000 in males) are reported from Argentina, Brazil (Recife) and Jamaica. In Asia, high incidence rates are seen in most countries except India and Israel. Over 30 per 100,000 in males reported in China, Hong Kong, Japan (Osaka) and Singapore (Chinese). In Africa, a very high rate (>30 per 100,000 in males) is seen in Mozambique. A relatively high rate is seen in South Africa (28.4) and in Senegal (25.6). In Oceania, two populations reported high rate, the Melanesians in New Caledonia (18.7) and residents of Polynesian island in New Zealand. However, the actual rates are not as high as those registered in Asia or Africa. In North America, high rates are observed among ethnic groups migrating from high-risk countries from China, Korea and Japan. Black Americans have a consistently high incidence rate, 2 to 3 times higher than white Americans. Although there are a few reports on the relationship between non-A, non-B hepatitis and HCC in the United States [5–7], it appears that hepatitis virus-related HCC is found much less frequently in the United States than in Asia, Africa and South Europe. In Canada, the population of Eskimos indicates a high rate (6.9 in male) but not in Alberta (1.3 in male) [5].

With practically no geographic exception, HCC is more common in males than in females, but the male/female ratio differs with the country as well as with the year of survey because of changing time trends. It appears that the male/female ratio is greater in the high-prevalence regions, such as Africa, China and Japan; but lower in the low-incidence regions, such as Europe and South America.

It is well known that the mean age of patients with HCC is different between hepatitis B virus (HBV)-related and HCV-related HCC. In Japan the mean age of HBV-related HCC is around 50 years, and of HCV-related HCC is around 63 years [8–10]. This discrepancy may depend on the initial infection time of HBV and HCV. HBV infection occurs in neonatal (mainly maternal transmission), and HCV infection occurs in adolescence.

Epidemiology of HCC in Japan

According to vital statistics of Japan 1993 [11], the mortality of patients with HCC has increased dramatically over the last 20 years. HCC is the third leading cause of death among men suffering from cancer, and approximately 30,000 patients in Japan died of HCC in 1993 [11].

In an analysis of Osaka Cancer Registry data, Okuda et al. [12] reported that the annual incidence of primary liver cancer in men in the Osaka area, where chronic liver disease is most prevalent in Japan, was 16.3 per 100,000 from 1966 to 1968, and 40.9 per 100,000, a record 2-fold increase, from 1984 to 1986. From 1958 to 1959, HCC constituted 5.78% of all malignancies, but by 1982 the relative incidence had increased to 14.0%, representing more than a 2-fold increase. Recent statistics reported by the Japanese Ministry of Health and Welfare indicate that the mortality due to HCC in men is much higher than that in women, also that HCC is the first leading cause of death in men aged between 50 and 60 years (Fig. 1).

The geographical distribution by Japanese prefecture of corrected mortality rates for HCC shows a gradient, with the incidence being higher in the West than in the East [8]. HBV and HCV infections are major causative agents of HCC in Japan. The prevalence of hepatitis B surface antigen (HBsAg) and of

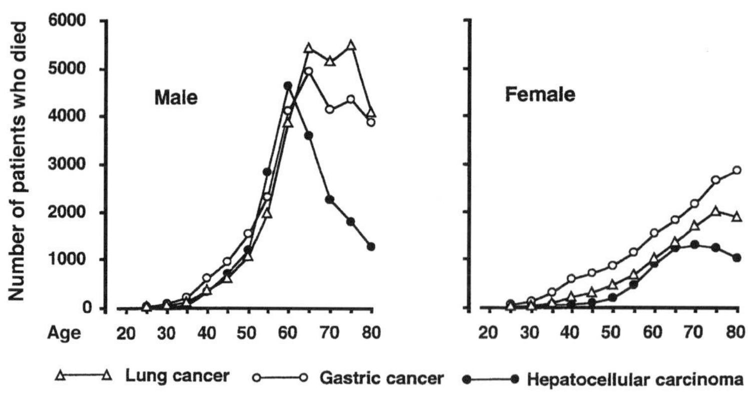

Fig. 1. Age-adjusted mortality rates for hepatocellular cancer, lung cancer and gastric cancer. Right: male, Left: female (1993 statistics from the Japanese Ministry of Health and Welfare).

antibody to hepatitis C virus (anti-HCV) among blood donors is higher in the West than in the East, and both gradients are parallel to that of HCC.

HBV- and HCV-related HCC worldwide

HCC is frequently associated with chronic HBV and HCV infection, and both viruses are believed to be causative factors in a large percentage of cases. In geographic regions where HBV and HCV are endemic, such as in Africa, Asia and Mediterranean regions, HCC is common. In geographic regions where HBV and HCV are not endemic, such as North America and north Europe, HCC is uncommon.

The prevalence of anti-HCV and HBsAg in patients with HCC worldwide is shown in Table 2. A high prevalence of anti-HCV has been observed in patients with HBsAg-negative HCC in Italy (70–79%) [13–16], Spain (77%) [17] and Japan (75–90%) [2,18,19]. A relatively high prevalence has been observed in France (57%) [20], Florida, USA (49%) [21], and low prevalence in Germany (16%) [22], India (9%) [23], Bangladesh (8%) [24], Taiwan (23% [25], 10% [26],

Table 2. Prevalence (%) HBV-related and HCV-related HCC worldwide.

Region	HBsAg / anti-HCV (%)				
	n	+/–	–/+	+/+	–/–
Europe					
Italy, Lerrero [16]	167	23	49	9	19
Colombo [13]	132	14	51	17	18
Simmonetti [14]	212	7	62	9	22
Spain, Bruix [17]	88	25	72	0	3
France, Nalpas [20]	55	6	58	16	20
Germany, Goeser [22]	81	36	16	12	36
Africa					
South Africa, Kew [29]	380	36	16	12	36
Asia					
Saudi Arabia, Ali [32]	42	33	26	5	36
India, Mamesh [23]	53	23	9	6	62
Thailand, Boonmar [33]	47	60	38	2	0
Hong Kong, Leung [28]	424	80	4	4	12
Taiwan, Chen [25]	66	55	23	11	13
Chung [26]	128	68	10	9	13
Lee [27]	326	72	9	3	16
Japan, Kiyosawa [2]	83	23	61	12	4
Nishioka [18]	180	36	44	6	14
Nepal, Shrestha	62	39	14	0	47
Bangladesh, Khan [24]	50	44	8	0	48
North America					
USA,Yu [30]	51	20	9	18	53
DiBisceglie [31]	99	7	12	1	80

9% [27]), Hong Kong (7%) [28] and South Africa (16%) [29]. The prevalence of HBV-related HCC was less than 10% in the USA, and that of HCV-related HCC 13—30% [30,31]. In Europe, the prevalence of HBV-related and HCV-related HCC were respectively, 23% and 49% in north Italy [16], 7% and 62% in south Italy [15], 25% and 72% in Spain [17]. In Taiwan [25—27], South Africa [29], Saudi Arabia [32] and Thailand [33], the prevalence of HBV-related HCC was higher than that of HCV related one. In Japan, the prevalence of HCV-related HCC was much higher than that of HBV-related HCC [2,18]. It is noted that, HCV- and HBV-non-related HCC is seen as a relatively high proportion in Asian countries.

Chronological changes in HBV- and HCV-related HCC between 1971 and 1994

As mentioned above, the number of patients with HCC in Japan steadily increased [34]. To clarify the chronological changes in hepatitis virus types in HCC cases, 541 patients with HCC who were treated at Shinshu University Hospital and its affiliated hospitals between 1971 and 1995 were analyzed for HBsAg and anti-HCV (Table 3). There were 112 patients in 1971—1980, 267 in 1981—1990, and 162 in 1991—1995. The ratio of men to women was 5.2 for 1971—1980, 5.4 for 1981—1990, and 1.9 for 1991—1995. These data indicate that the incidence of HCC has increased rapidly not only in men but also in women.

The prevalence of each type of HCC, HBV-related HCC patients was 54%, 31% and 13% in 1971—1980, 1981—1990 and 1991—1995, respectively. On the contrary, the prevalence of HCV-related HCC patients was 34%, 59% and 79%, in 1971—1980, 1981—1990 and 1991—1995, respectively. Unclassified patients were presented 5 ∼ 8% in each period. These findings clearly indicate that HCV-

Table 3. Number of patients with HCC of each hepatitis viral type between 1971 and 1995 at Shinshu University Hospital.

Period	Total		HBsAg/anti-HCV							
			+/−		−/+		+/+		−/−	
	M	W	M	W	M	W	M	W	M	W
1971—1980	94	18	50	10	32	6	4	1	8	1
	112 (100%)		60 (54%)		38 (34%)		5 (4%)		9 (8%)	
1981—1990	225	42	72	10	128	31	4	0	21	1
	267 (100%)		82 (31%)		159 (59%)		4 (2%)		22 (8%)	
1991—1995	106	56	17	4	79	49	4	1	6	2
	162 (100%)		21 (13%)		128 (79%)		5 (3%)		8 (5%)	

Note: M = men, W = women.

related HCC increased over the time trends. The reason for the increase in the number of patients with HCC in Japan might be the increase in chronic hepatitis C. This may have been inherited or passed on by a blood transfusion or caused by infection from a tattoo 20 to 40 years ago.

HCV genotype and HCC

According to a recent consensual nomenclature, HCV genetic variants are hierarchically classified into major groups (types) corresponding to the main branches of the viral phylogenetic tree and, within them, into more closely related subgroups (subtypes) [35]. Differences in HCV-genotype distribution have been documented in various countries. There have been several reports that HCV genotype (subtype) distribution may change significantly according to the histological severity of liver lesions and, in particular, that HCV type 1b is overrepresented among patients with advanced disease, such as cirrhosis and HCC [36—42]. Nousbaum et al. [38] conducted the cross-sectional study among French and Italian patients with HCV-related chronic liver disease. They postulated that HCV type 1b is highly prevalent among patients with severe liver disease. The prevalence was 84.8% in patients with both cirrhosis and hepatocellular carcinomas, 75.4% in patients with cirrhosis who did not have hepatocellular carcinoma, and only 53.8% in patients with chronic hepatitis. In contrast, HCV infections with type 1a alone, or with types 2a, 2b or 3a, were more frequently seen in patients with chronic hepatitis who did not have cirrhosis or hepatocellular carcinoma. This raises the possibility that HCV type 1b exerts a specific cytopathogenic effect. Silini et al. [41] also conducted a cross-sectional and a case-control analysis in 593 patients with chronic hepatitis C with or without HCC. They demonstrated that HCV 1b infection is more prevalent among patients with HCC compared with patients with cirrhosis but without HCC and chronic hepatitis. Though age, male sex, and HCV 1b influenced the risk of cancer in cirrhosis, by univariate analysis, HCV 1b was independently associated with HCC by a pair-wise comparison. Similar study has been performed by Tanaka et al. [43] in Japan. Sixteen medical institutions in Japan collaborated in this study of the epidemiology of HCV genotypes. A total of 4,176 patients with type C chronic liver disease, from the four main islands of Japan, were evaluated. Of those evaluated, 2,794 had chronic hepatitis, 727 had liver cirrhosis and 655 had hepatocellular carcinoma. The HCV genotype of the patients was determined by an enzyme-linked immunosorbent assay based on serological genotype 1- and 2-specific recombinant peptides (SG-1 and SG-2, respectively) of the NS4 region. The prevalence of SG-1 and SG-2 HCV was similar in the four main islands of Japan.

SG-1 HCV predominated in each disease category (69—76%). The percentage of patients with SG-1 HCV increased by 7%, while that of patients with SG-2 HCV decreased by 7%, as liver disease progressed in severity from chronic hepatitis to carcinoma ($p < 0.001$). Patients with either SG-1 or SG-2 had a similar mean age and history of blood transfusion. In conclusion, SG-1 HCV was found to predominate in Japan, and the HCV genotype was found to be related to the stage of hepatitis C disease.

Kobayashi et al. [42] compared the long-term histological outcome of chronic hepatitis infected with HCV genotype 1 (1a, 1b) and HCV genotype 2 (2a, 2b) to clarify the difference of pathogenicity between these genotypes. According to this, deteriorations of grading and staging were seen in 68 and 63% of the patients with genotype 1, respectively. On the contrary, deterioration rate was 41.7% in grading and 38.9% in staging of the patients with genotype 2. Risk factors related to the development of HCC were demonstrated to be not only the initial stage of liver histology, age and follow-up period but also HCV genotype 1. Bruno et al. [44] conducted the same study among patients with HCV-infected liver cirrhosis. A cohort of 163 consecutive patients was prospectively evaluated for the development HCC in each genotype. After 5- to 7-year follow-up (median, 68 months), HCC developed in 22 of the patients, 19 infected with type 1b and with type 2a/c ($p<0.005$). Multivariate analysis showed that type 1b was the most important risk factor associated with HCC development (odds ratio 6.14, 1.77–21.37, 95% confidence interval). This indicates that HCV 1b infected cirrhosis patients carry a significantly higher risk of developing HCC than patients infected by other HCV types. These observations give us very important information on how to follow HCV-infected liver cirrhosis patients.

References

1. Choo QL, Weiner AJ, Kuo G, Overby LR, Bradley DW, Houghton M. Isolation of cDNA clone derived form a blood-borne non-A, non-B viral hepatitis genome. Science 1989;244:359–362.
2. Kiyosawa K, Sodeyama T, Tanaka E, Gibo Y, Yoshizawa K, Nakano Y, Furuta S, Akahane Y, Nishioka K, Purcell RH, Alter HJ. Interrelationship of blood transfusion, non-A, non-B hepatitis and hepatocellular carcinoma: analysis by detection of antibody to hepatitis C virus. Hepatology 1990;12:671–675.
3. Sullivan D, Gerber MA. Conservation of hepatitis C virus 5′untranslated sequences in hepatocellular carcinoma and the surrounding liver. Hepatology 1994;19:551–553.
4. Yoshizawa K, Kiyosawa K, Usuda S, Yabu K, Nakatsuji Y, Yamada S, Tanaka E, Sodeyama T, Furuta S, Kaneko S, Nakane PK. New hepatocellular carcinoma cell line SUHC-1 established from a patient with hepatitis C virus RNA in serum. Jpn J Cancer Res 1992;83:871–877.
5. Bosh FX, Munoz N. Hepatocelluar carcinoma in the world: epidemiologic questions. In: Tabor E, Di Bisceglie AM, Purcell RH (eds) Etiology, Pathology, and Treatment of Hepatocelluar Carcinoma in North America. Woodlands: Portfolio Publishing Company, Houston: Gulf Publishing Company, 1991:35–54(199).
6. Cohen EB, Gang DL, Zeldis JB. Primary hepatocellular carcinoma following nonspecific non-B hepatitis with tumor DNA negative for HBV DNA. Dis Dis Sci 32;1428–1430,1987.
7. Gilliam JH, Geisinger KR, Zeldis JB. Primary hepatocellular carcinoma after chronic non-A, non-B posttransfusion hepatitis. Ann Intern Med 1984;101:797–795.
8. Kiyosawa K, Furuta A. Clinical aspects and epidemiology of hepatitis B and C viruses in hepatocellular carcinoma in Japan. Can Chemot Pharm 1992;31:S150–S156.
9. Shiratori Y, Shiina S, Imamura M, Kato N, Kanai F, Okudaira T, Teratani T, Tohgo G, Toda N, Ohashi M, Ogura K, Niwa Y, Kawabe T, Omata M. Characteristic difference of hepatocellular carcinoma. Hepatology 1995;22:1027–1033.

10. Miyagawa S, Kawasaki S, Makuuchi M. Comparison of the characteristics of hepatocellular carcinoma between hepatitis B and C viral infection; Tumor multicentricity in cirrhotic liver with hepatitis C. Hepatology 1996;24:307–310.
11. Vital Statistics 1992 Japan. Statics and Information Department, Minister's Secretariat, Ministry of Health & Wefare.
12. Okuda K, Fujimoto I, Hanai A, Urano Y. Changing incidence of hepatocellular carcinoma in Japan. Cancer Res 1987;47:4967–4972.
13. Colombo M, Kuo G, Choo QL, Donato MF, Del Ninno E, Tommasini MA, Diuguardi N, Houghton M. Prevalence of antibodies to hepatitis C virus in Italian patients with hepatocellular carcinoma. Lancet 1989;ii:1006–1008.
14. Simmonetti RG, Cottone M, Craxi A, Pagliaro L, Rapicetta M, Chionne P, Constantino A. Prevalence of antibodies to hepatitis C virus in hepatocellular carcinoma. Lancet 1989;ii:1338.
15. Simmonetti RG, Camma CC, Fiorello F, Cottone M, Rapicetta M, Marino L, Firorentino G, Craxi A, Ciccaglione A, Giuseppetti R, Stroffolini T, Pagliaro L. Hepatitis C virus infections as a risk for hepatocellular carcinoma in patients with cirrhosis. A case-control study. Ann Intern Med 1992;116:97–102.
16. Levrero M, Tagger A, Balsano C, De Marizio E, Avvantaggiati ML, Natoli G, Diop D, Villa E, Diodati G, Alberti A. Antibodies to hepatitis C virus in patients with hepatocellular carcinoma. J Hepatol 1991;12:60–63.
17. Bruix J, Barrera JM, Cavet X, Ercilla G, Costa T, Sanchez-Tapias JM, Vantura M, Vall M, Bruguera M, Bru C, Castillo R, Rodes J. Prevalence of antibodies to hepatitis C virus in Spanish patients with hepatocellular carcinoma and hepatic cirrhosis. Lancet 1989;ii:1004–1006.
18. Nishioka K, Watanabe J, Furuta S, Tanaka E, Iino S, Suzuki H, Tsuji T, Yano M, Kuo G, Choo QL, Houghton M, Oda T. A high prevalence of antibody to hepatitis C virus in patients with hepatocellular carcinoma in Japan. Cancer 1991;67:429–433.
19. Saito I, Miyamura T, Ohbayashi A, Choo QL, Kuo G, Houghton M. Hepatitis C virus infection is associated with the development of hepatocellular carcinoma. Proc Natl Acad Sci USA 1990;87:6547–6549.
20. Nalpas B, Driss F, Pol S, Hamelin B, Housset C, Brechot C, Berthelot P. Association between HCV and HBV infection in hepatocellular carcinoma and alcoholic liver diseas. J Hepatol 1991;12:70–74.
21. Hasan F, Jeffers LJ, De Medina M, Reddy KR, Parker T, Shiff E, Houghton M, Choo QL, Kuo G. Hepatitis C-associated hepatocellular carcinoma. Hepatology 1990;12:589–591.
22. Goeser T, Muller HM, Solbach C et al. Hepatitis C virus, alcoholic cirrhosis and hepatocellular carcinoma. Cancer Epidemiol Biomar Prev 1994;3:311–315.
23. Ramesh R, Munshi A, Panda SK. Prevalence of hepatitis C virus antibodies in chronic liver disease and hepatocellular carcinoma patients in India. J Gastroenterol Hepatol 1992:7:393–395.
24. Khan M, Ahmad N. Seroepidemiology of HBG and HCV in Bangradesh. Intern Hepatol Commu 1996;5:27–29.
25. Chen DS, Kuo G, Sung JL, Lai MY, Sheu JC, Chen PJ, Yang PM, Hsu HM, Chang MH, Chen CJ, Hahn LC, Choo QL, Wang TH, Houghton M. Prevalence of anti-HCV in patients with hepatocellular carcinoma in Taiwan. J Infect Dis 1990;162:817–822.
26. Chung WL, Chang WY, Lu SN, Su WP, Lin ZY, Chen SC, Heieh MY, Wang LY, You SL, Chen CJ. The role of hepatitis B and C viruses in hepatocellular carcinoma in a hepatitis B endemic area: case control study. Cancer 1992;69:2052–2054.
27. Lee SD, Lee FY, Wu JC, Hwang AJ, Wang SS, Juei KJ. The prevalence of anti-hepatitis C virus among Chinese patients with hepatocellular carcinoma. Cancer 1991;69:342–345.
28. Leung NWY, Tam JS, Lai JY, Leung TWT, Lau WY, Shin W, Li AK. Does hepatitis C virus infection contribute to hepatocellular carcinoma? Cancer 1992;70:40–44.
29. Kew MC, Houghton M, Choo QL, Kuo G. Hepatitis C virus antibodies in southern African blacks with hepatocellular carcinoma. Lancet 1990;i:873–874.
30. Yu MC, Tong MJ, Cousaget P, Ross PK, Govindalajan S, Henderson BE. Prevalence of hepatitis

B and C viral markers in black and white patients with hepatocellular carcinoma in the United States. J Natl Cancer Inst 1990;82:1038–1041.
31. Di Bisceglie AM, Order SE, Klein L, Waggoner LG, Sjogren WH, Kuo G, Houghton M, Choo QL, Hoofnagle JH. The role of chronic viral hepatitis in hepatocellular carcinoma in the United States Am J Gastroenterol 1991;86:335–338.
32. Ali M, Shapiro S, Rahman A, Mohamed RES, Asfeed AA, Ahmed AMM. Hepatitis C virus infection in chronic liver disease and hepatocellular carcinoma in Saudi Arabia. J Hepatogastroenterol Hepatol 1992;27:237–239.
33. Boonmar S, Pojanagaroon B, Watanabe Y, Tanaka Y, Miyamura T. Prevalence of hepatitis C virus antibody among healthy blood donors and non-A, non-B hepatitis patients in Thailand. Jpn J Med Sci Biol 1990;43:29–36.
34. Furuta K, Kiyosawa K, Sone H, Matsumoto A, Tanaka E, Sodeyama T, Imai H, Furuta S. Chronological changes of hepatitis B and C virus markers in Japanese patients with hepatocellular carcinoma. In: Nishioka K, Suzuki H, Mishiro S, Oda T (eds) Viral Hepatitis and Liver Disease. Tokyo: Springer-Verlag, 1994,690–693.
35. Simmonds P. Variability of hepatitis C virus. Hepatology 1995;21:570–583.
36. Silini EM, Bono F, Cividini A, Cerino A, Bruno S, Rossi S, Belloni G, Brugnetti B, Civardi E, Salvaneschi L, Mondelli MU. Differential distribution of hepatitis C virus genotypes in patients with and wothout liver function abnormalities. Hepatology 1995;21:285–290.
37. Pozzato G, Kaneko S, Moretti M, Croce LS, Franzin F, Unoura M, Bercich L, tribelli C, Crovatto M, Santini G, Kobayashi K. Different genotypes of hepatitis C virus are associated with different severity of chronic liver disease. J Med Virol 1994;43:291–296.
38. Nousbaum L-B, Pol S, Nalpas B, Landais P, Berthelot P, Brechot C. Hepatitis C virus type 1b(II) infection in France and Italy. Ann Intern Med 1995;122:111–120.
39. Silini E, Mondelli MU. The significance of HCV genotypes. Vir Hepatitis Rev 1995;1:111–120.
40. Silini E, Bono F, Cerino A, Piazza V, Solcia E, Mondelli MU. Virological features of hepatitis C virus infection in hemodialysis patients. J Clin Microbiol 1993;31:2913–2917.
41. Silini E, Bottelli R, Asti M, Bruno S, Candusso ME, Brambilla S, Bono F, Iamoni G, Tinelli C, Mondelli MU, Ideo G. Hepatitis C virus genotypes and risk of hepatocellular carcinoma in cirrhosis: a case control study. Gastroenterology 1996;111:199–205.
42. Kobayashi M, Tanaka E, Sodeyama T, Urushihara A, Matsumoto A, Kiyosawa K. The natural course of chronic hepatitis C: a comparison between patients with genotypes 1 and 2 hepatitis C viruses. Hepatology 1996;23:695–699.
43. Tanaka E, Kiyosawa K, Matsushima T, Ishikawa K, Hino K, Tanaka S, Nose H, Kumada H, Iino S, Kamimura T, Uniura M, Mizokami M, Okanoue T, Kuroki T, Yamada G, Miura T, Yano M, Tsubouchi H, Kohara M, Sato S, Hattori N, Genotyping ELISA Study Group. J Gastroenterol Hepatol 1995;10:538–545.
44. Bruno S, Silini E, Crosignani et al. Hepatitis C virus and risk of hepatocellular carcinoma in cirrhosis: a prospective study. Hepatology 1997;25:754–758.

Progress in Hepatology, Volume 3.
Hepatocellular Carcinoma.
M. Yamanaka, G. Toda and T. Tanaka, editors.

Pathology of early hepatocellular carcinoma

Masamichi Kojiro
First Department of Pathology, Kurume University School of Medicine, Kurume, Japan

Abstract. According to the extensive studies on small hepatocellular carcinomas (HCC) in an early stage in the past decade, the pathomorphologic features of early HCC have been clarified. In general, early HCCs are classified into two major forms: distinctly nodular type and vaguely nodular type. The latter consists of uniform distribution of well-differentiated cancerous tissues and contains portal tracts. The most characteristic feature of early HCC is that the majority of them are well-differentiated. Well-differentiated HCCs in an early stage are characterized by the following features; i) increased cell density with irregular thin-trabecular pattern, ii) frequent acinar and/or pseudoglandular pattern, iii) frequent fatty change. In addition, coexistence of more than two cancerous tissues with different histologic grade is common in small HCCs up to 2 cm in diameter, and some of them show "nodule-in-nodule" appearance, macroscopically. Such a "nodule-in-nodule" appearance seems to reflect the progression of dedifferentiation phenomenon in well-differentiated HCCs.

Keywords: early hepatocellular carcinoma, liver cirrhosis, nodule-in-nodule, pathology, small liver cancer, well-differentiated hepatocellular carcinoma.

Underlying liver cirrhosis

It is well known that more than 80% of hepatocellular carcinoma (HCC) occur in cirrhotic liver. Recently, it has been clarified that the morphologic features are significantly different among hepatitis B virus (HBV)-related and hepatitis C virus (HCV)-related cirrhosis [1]. In Japan, HCC has been steeply increasing since 1975. This is a result of an increase in HCV-related cases [2]. Namely, according to the nationwide survey of HCC by Liver Cancer Study Group of Japan, 40.7% of HCC were positive to hepatitis B surface antigen (HBsAg) in the period of 10 years from 1968 to 1977, but only 17.8% were HBsAg-positive in the period from 1990 to 1991 [3]. It is predicted that such a remarkable trend in the prevalence of hepatitis virus related to HCC in the past 25 years might be reflected in the morphology of liver cirrhosis associated with HCC.

HBV-related liver cirrhosis (type B cirrhosis) with HCC

The morphological characteristics of type B cirrhosis bearing HCC are characterized by the following features: 1) finely expanding fibrous septa and large regenerative nodules; 2) weak inflammatory reaction and little piecemeal necrosis; 3) marked regenerative activity of the hepatocytes with frequent liver cell dysplasia

Address for correspondence: Masamichi Kojiro MD, First Department of Pathology, Kurume University School of Medicine, Kurume 830, Japan. Fax: +81-942-32-0905.

of Anthony [4]. Generally, type B cirrhosis shows the features of macronodular cirrhosis (Fig. 1A). Histologically, active inflammation with piecemeal necrosis is not remarkable. In the parenchyma, marked regenerative activity of hepatocytes showing a cobblestone arrangement with liver cell dysplasia is common (Fig. 2A). The formation of large regenerative nodules in type B cirrhosis can be explained by active hepatocyte regeneration after subsidence of active inflammation following seroconversion. Although macronodular cirrhosis was associated with about 50% of HCCs until mid-1970s, it is now only a small percentage among autopsy cases. However, in Korea, Taiwan and Hong Kong where many of HCCs are closely related to HBV, association of macronodular cirrhosis is still common.

HCV antibody-positive liver cirrhosis (type C cirrhosis) bearing HCC

The morphological features of type C cirrhosis are characterized by the following features: 1) small and irregular shaped regenerative nodules (Fig. 1B); 2) relatively strong inflammatory reaction with frequent lymphoid aggregation and frequent lymphoid follicle formation (Fig. 2B). These characteristic features are

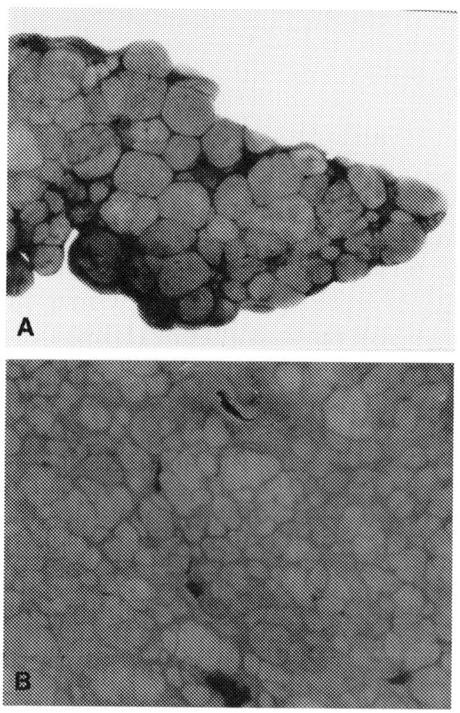

Fig. 1. Gross features of HBV-related and HCV-related liver cirrhosis. **A**: HBV-related liver cirrhosis is composed of large and regular shaped regenerative nodules. **B**: HCV-related cirrhosis consists of small and irregular shaped regenerative nodules.

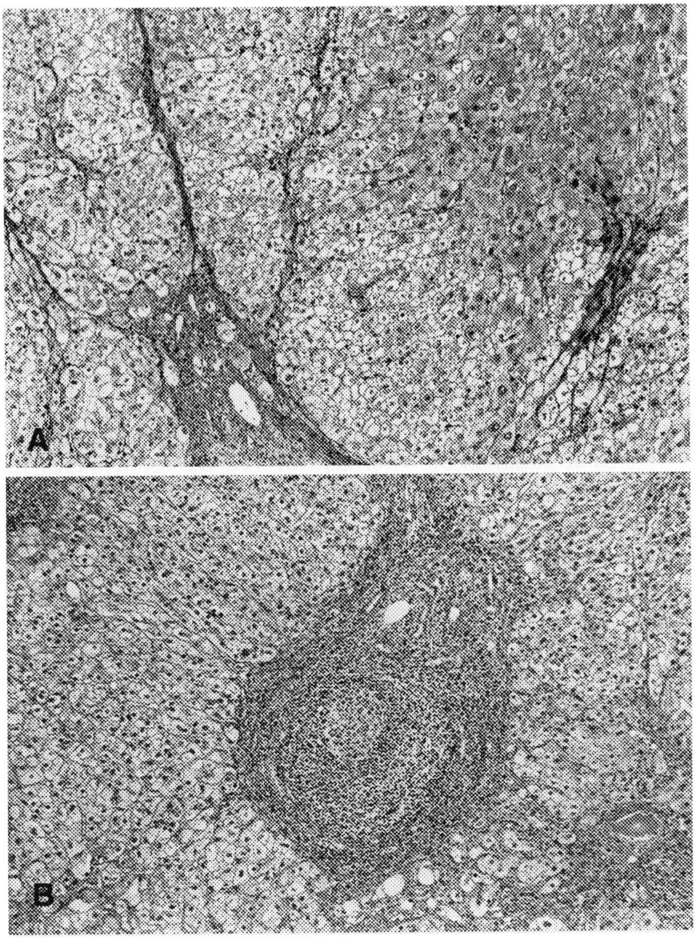

Fig. 2. Histologic features of HBV-related and HCV-related liver cirrhosis. **A**: In HBV-related liver cirrhosis, hepatocytes show active regenerative features with liver cell dysplasia of Anthony and little active inflammation. **B**: In HCV-related cirrhosis, active inflammation with lymphoid follicle formation and piecemeal necrosis of liver parenchyma is dominant.

most appreciable in surgical cases, and many of type C cirrhosis cannot be classified by conventional gross classifications for liver cirrhosis. It is of great interest that type C cirrhosis, in comparison with type B, shows stronger inflammatory reactions associated with piecemeal necrosis along the fibrous septa. The definite cause of such marked inflammatory reactions in type C cirrhosis is not known, but it has been considered to be related to continuous replication of HCV in hepatocytes. Such active inflammation in type C cirrhosis might reflect viral replication and immune reaction in liver tissue. Replication of HBV has been reported to decrease along with the progression of disease, while the number of virus copies in serum is low but gradually increases in hepatitis C patients.

The histometrical analysis of surgical cases of liver cirrhosis associated with HCC disclosed a significant difference in the size of regenerative nodules and the area of fibrous septum among type B and type C cirrhosis; namely, the average size of regenerative nodules in type B cirrhosis (40.5 ± 22.7 (SD) mm) is approximately 3 times larger than 16.9 ± 10.8 (SD) mm of type C cirrhosis. It is likely that persistent active inflammatory reaction in type C cirrhosis may not allow for formation of large regenerative nodules. However, strong regenerative activity after subsidence of inflammatory reaction following seroconversion does lead to formation of large regenerative nodules in type B cirrhosis.

Chronological trends in the morphologic type of liver cirrhosis associated with HCC

HCC is steeply increasing since around 1975, and the cause of such a steep increase has been explained by a remarkable increase of HCV-related cases in Japan. Until about 2 decades ago, approximately 30—40% of HCC were positive to HBsAg in Japan, but it is only less than 10% at present and approximately 80% of HCC are positive to anti-HCV. Thus, it is suggested that such prominent chronological trends of hepatitis virus related to HCC may be reflected in the morphology of liver cirrhosis associated with HCC. In the morphologic comparison of liver cirrhosis associated with HCC in the 6 years period from 1970 to 1975 before the epidemiological analysis disclosed a steep increase of HCC and those in the 6 years period from 1989 to 1994, a significant difference was observed. Among 67 liver cirrhosis associated with HCC from 1970 to 1975, 26 (38.8%) were of macronodular type which is characterized by large regenerative nodules 5—10 mm in diameter and relatively thin-fibrous septa; 35 (52.2%) were of mixed macro- and micronodular type consisting of a varying mixture of small and large regenerative nodules, and one was of micronodular type. HBsAg was positive in 57.1% of the macronodular type and 22.2% of the mixed type examined. On the other hand, among 44 hepatocellular carcinoma cases from 1989 to 1994, macronodular cirrhosis was found only in six (13.6%), and four (66.7%) of them were positive to HBsAg. Thirty-seven cases (84.1%) were of mixed macro- and micronodular type. Fifteen (93.8%) of 16 mixed type examined were positive to HCV antibody and only one (5.3%) of 19 mixed type examined was positive to HBsAg. Six were micronodular type without a history of alcohol abuse. Thus, it can be said that a prominent morphologic trend in liver cirrhosis associated HCC in the past 25 years truly reflects the chronological trends in hepatitis virus B and C which are the most pathogenic to HCC in Japan [5].

Comparison of HCC associated with type B cirrhosis and HCC with type C cirrhosis

Although a significant difference is not observed in tumor morphology itself, there is a significant difference in age and tumor size among surgical cases of HCCs with type B cirrhosis (B-related HCC) and those with type C cirrhosis (C-related HCC) [6].

The tumor size ranged from 1.5 to 11.5 cm with a mean of 4.5 ± 2.7(SD) cm in B-related HCCs and it ranged from 0.7 to 15.1 cm with a mean of 3.1 ± 1.9(SD) cm in C-related HCCs. The mean tumor size of the former is significantly larger than the latter. The frequency of the tumors less than 3.0 cm in diameter is 65% in C-related HCCs, but it is only 28% in B-related HCCs. There are two possible explanations for such a significant difference in the tumor size among both groups. Firstly, a minute HCC is less detectable in HBV-related liver cirrhosis which is composed of larger regenerative nodules. Recently, diagnostic imaging, in particular ultrasonography has become remarkably advanced, and periodic ultrasonographic examinations have become the most reliable means for detecting a minute HCC. In HBV-related cirrhosis, however, a minute tumor nodule may be concealed by the large regenerative nodules and may be difficult to detect until the tumor reaches a certain size much larger than the regenerative nodules. In contrast, as the regenerative nodules are much smaller in HCV-related cirrhosis, a minute tumor can be detected more easily. Secondly, the patients with HCV-related cirrhosis tend to visit the physicians more frequently than those with HBV-related cirrhosis because the former tend to have more deteriorated liver functions. Accordingly, they may have more chances of having an imaging examination.

Another distinct difference is that there is a significant difference in the average age among the two groups. For comparison, in 35 resected B-related HCCs and in 100 resected C-related HCCs, the mean age is 50.6 ± 9.9 (SD) years and 64.3 ± 7.3 (SD) years, respectively. Such a significant difference in average age may be explained by the different routes of virus transmission. Namely, perinatal and mother-to-infant infections are common sources in HBV carriers, whereas HCV is mainly transmitted by blood transfusions, dialysis, intravenous drug abuse, and so on, generally occurring in young adults.

Pathomorphologic characteristics of early hepatocellular carcinoma

General characteristics

Small HCC less than 2 cm in diameter can be categorized either into the distinct nodular type or vaguely nodular type [7]. Many of resected small HCCs ranging from 1.5 to 2.0 cm in diameter are the distinct nodular type, which presents a clear nodule with a fibrous capsule and/or fibrous septa (Fig. 3). On the other hand, the majority of vaguely nodular type are less than 1.5 cm in diameter (Fig. 4). Early HCCs of the vaguely nodular type consist of uniform distribution of well-differentiated cancerous tissues and contain portal tracts inside. Although most tumors in this category can be clearly detected either as a hypoechoic or hyperechoic nodular lesion in ultrasound examination, they are badly demarcated and it is occasionally difficult to distinguish them from the surrounding cirrhotic liver. Such an indistinctness of the tumor nodules is caused by the fact that they retain the basic architecture of the background cirrhotic liver due to a

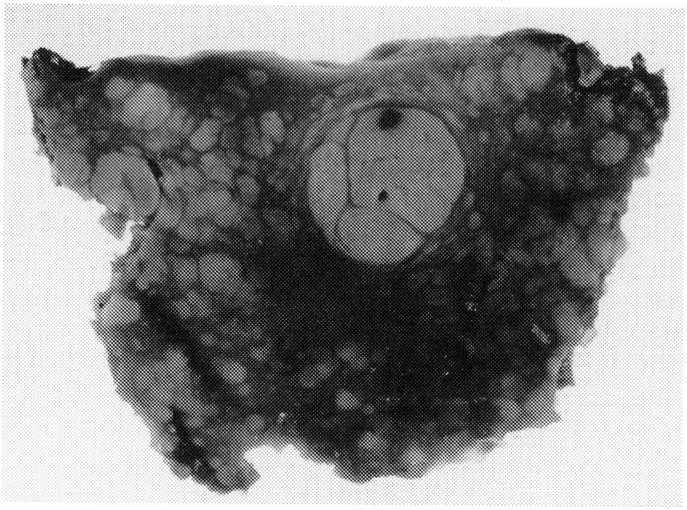

Fig. 3. Small hepatocellular carcinoma of distinctly nodular type. Thin fibrous capsule and septum are remarkable.

replacing growth of well-differentiated cancerous tissues. These findings are considered to be the characteristics of the smallest HCC which is clinically detectable at this moment.

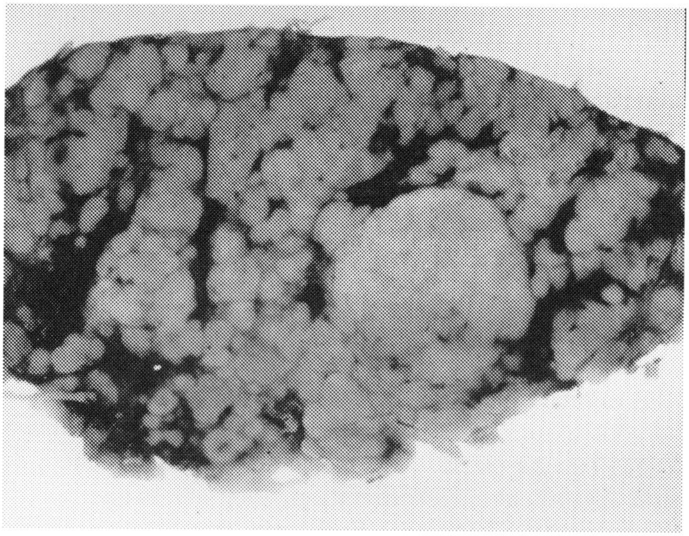

Fig. 4. Small hepatocellular carcinoma of vaguely nodular type. The tumor is vaguely nodular, and the tumor margin is indistinct.

Histologic characteristics

The most striking characteristic of early HCCs is that the majority of them are well-differentiated and well-differentiated hepatocellular carcinoma of vaguely nodular type often contains portal tracts [8,9] (Fig. 5). Cancer cells are arranged in a 2—3 cell thick plate and show an irregularly meandering thin-trabecular pattern. Sinusoid-like blood spaces are occasionally dilated, and/or are obscure due to swollen cancer cells. Increased cell density with increased nucleus/cytoplasm (N/C) ratio is also characteristic to well-differentiated HCC of the early stage. Increased cell density can be easily recognized by comparing the noncancerous tissue even in low power-field observation. The comparative observation of cancerous tissue and noncancerous tissue is inevitable in biopsy diagnosis of well-differentiated HCC with little atypia (Fig. 6). In general, cell density in well-differentiated HCC is more than 2 times that of noncancerous tissue. Along with a dedifferentiation of well-differentiated HCC to moderately or poorly differentiated HCC, cancer cells increase cell size and the cell density decreases. Generally, HCC cells have abundant eosinophilic cytoplasms. Although acinar and/or pseudoglandular pattern have been well known as one of the common features in HCC, those features are found in about 60% of well-differentiated HCCs of the early stage (Fig. 7). However, pseudoglandular pattern seen in well-differentiated HCCs is generally smaller than those in moderately differentiated HCCs, and many of them are found as acinar structure. Fatty change of cancer cells is also characteristic in early HCC [10] (Fig. 8). Varying degrees of fatty change are observed in 42.4% among the tumors ranging from 1.1 to 1.5 cm in diameter, and it is found only in 15.5% in the tumors larger than 3 cm in diameter. Fatty change in the tumors larger than 3 cm in diameter is seen only in part of the

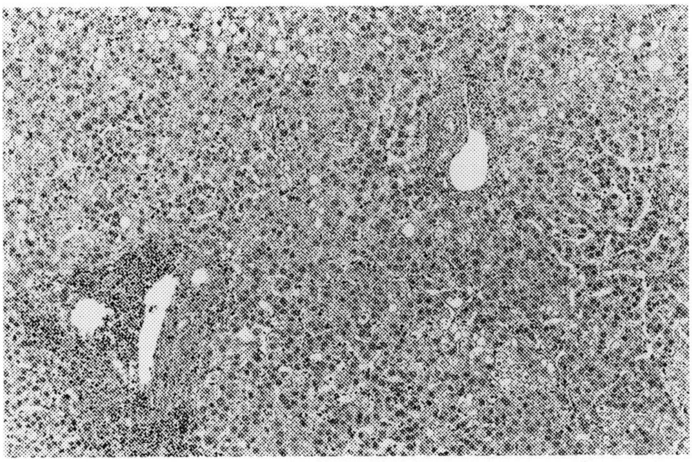

Fig. 5. Well-differentiated HCC containing portal tracts. The cancer cells are arranged in an irregular thin-trabecular pattern with focal fatty change. This feature is common in early HCCs of vaguely nodular type.

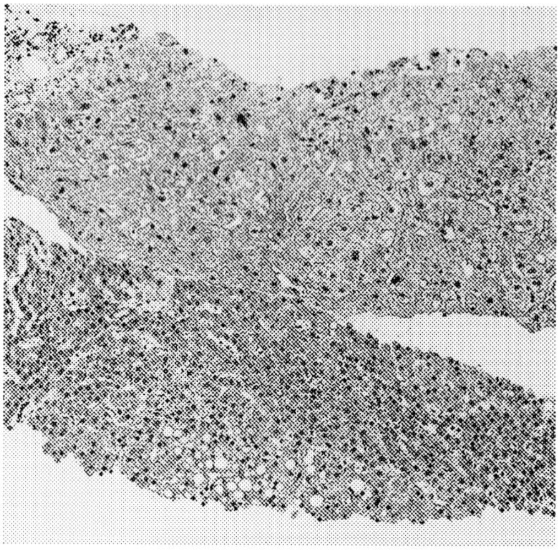

Fig. 6. Biopsy specimen of well-differentiated HCC cancer (lower specimen) is clearly identified by comparing with noncancerous tissue (above specimen).

tumor. In tumors with diffuse fatty change, diagnosis of HCC is sometimes difficult even in the resected specimens, and it is more difficult in biopsy specimens.

Coexistence of cancerous tissues with different histologic grade and different histologic type

Among the histologic varieties seen in early HCCs, the coexistence of cancerous tissues with different histologic grade is frequently observed [11] (Fig. 9). When

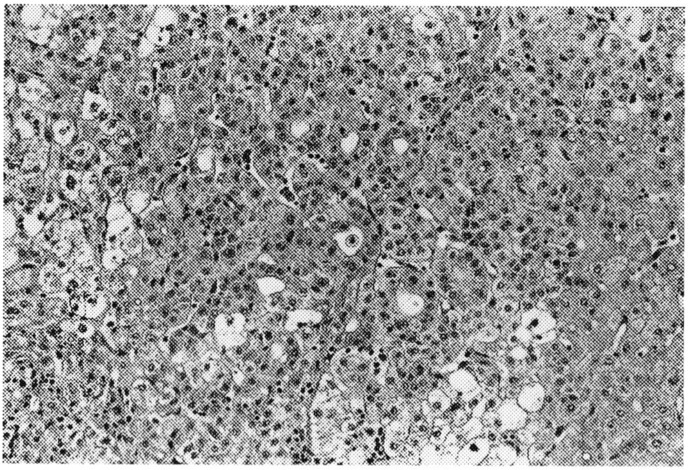

Fig. 7. Well-differentiated HCC with pseudoglandular structure. Cancer cells are arranged in an irregular thin-trabecular pattern with occasional pseudogland formation.

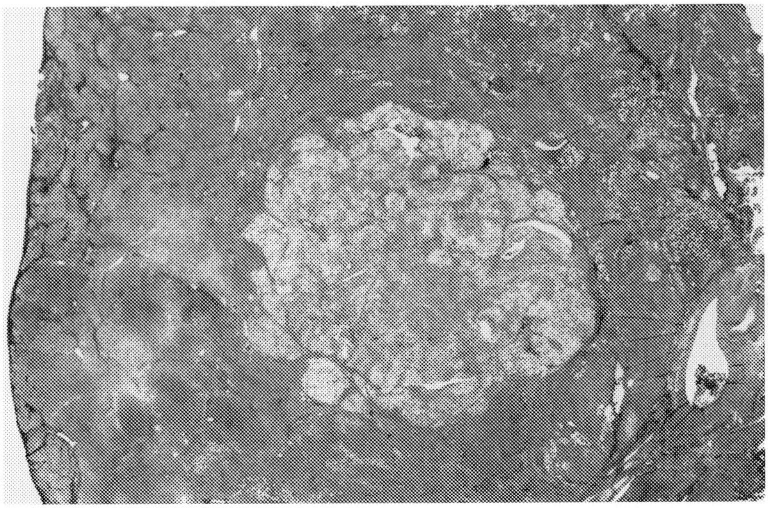

Fig. 8. Small HCC with diffuse fatty change. The tumor is found as a lucent tumor due to diffuse fatty change.

well-differentiated HCCs reach to around 1.5 cm in diameter, moderately or poorly differentiated cancerous tissues develop within the tumor. In such HCC nodules, moderately or poorly differentiated cancerous tissues are always located inside, and the well-differentiated one is located outside. The areas of well-differentiated cancerous tissues diminish in size along with an increase of the tumor size. The variety in histologic grade in early HCC nodules is considered to reflect a close correlation between tumor dedifferentiation and proliferation. When

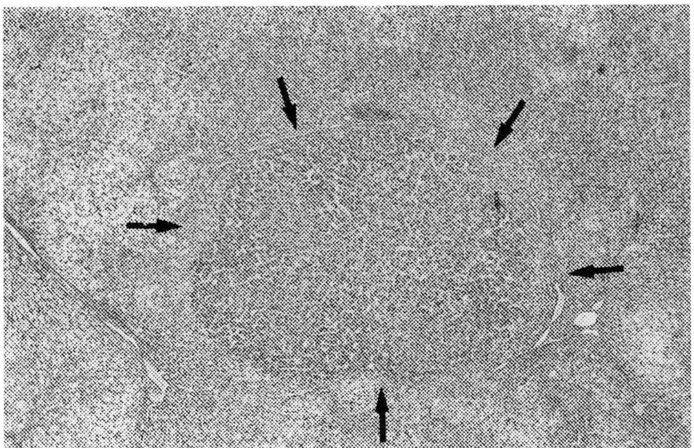

Fig. 9. Clear presence of moderately differentiated cancerous tissue (arrows) in a well-differentiated HCC.

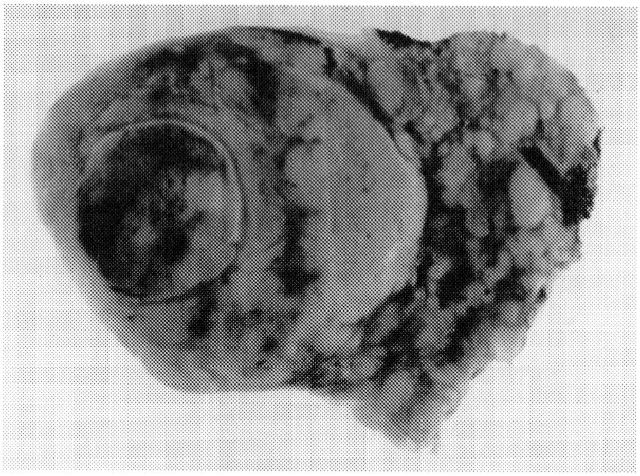

Fig. 10. Small HCC showing a typical "nodule in nodule" appearance.

HCC tumors contain a well-demarcated tumor nodule inside, it is called "nodule-in-nodule" appearance (Fig. 10). "Nodule-in-nodule" appearance is clearly appreciable by ultrasonography and its demonstration is considered to be diagnostic to HCC. Histologically, when HCC tumor contains a well-demarcated tumor tissue with different histologic features, the tumor tends to show a "nodule-in-nodule" appearance. In general, the most typical "nodule-in-nodule" appearance is appreciable in well-differentiated tumor containing less-differentiated tumor nodule with an expansive growth. This feature can be considered as the morphologic reflection of the dedifferentiation of well-differentiated HCC. Further, it has been clarified that dedifferentiation of well-differentiated HCC to less-differentiated HCC is a monoclonal phenomenon [12].

References

1. Shimamatsu K, Kage M, Nakashima O, Kojiro M. Pathomorphological study of HCV antibody positive liver cirrhosis. J Gastroenterol Hepatol 1994;9:624–630.
2. Kiyosawa K, Furuta S. Review of hepatitis C in Japan. J Gastroenterol Hepatol 1991;6:383–391.
3. Liver Cancer Study Group of Japan. Report of the 11th nationwide analysis of primary liver cancers (1990–1991), 1993. (in Japanese.)
4. Anthony PP. Primary carcinoma of the liver; a study of 282 cases of Uganda Africans. J Pathol 1973;1101:37–48.
5. Kojiro M. Hepatocellular carcinoma in hepatitis B virus-related and hepatitis C virus-related liver cirrhosis. In: Okita K (ed) Hepatology in '95. Japan:Axel Springer, 1995:11–20.
6. Takazawa T, Nakashima O, Sueda J, Tanaka M, Kojiro M. Clinicopathologic comparison of hepatitis B virus-related and hepatitis C virus-related hepatocellular carcinoma. Int J Oncol 1996;9:705–709.
7. Nakashima O, Sugihara S, Kage M. Pathomorphologic characteristics of small hepatocellular carcinoma: a special reference to small hepatocellular carcinoma with indistinct margins. Hepatology 1995;22:101–105.

8. Kondo Y, Niwa Y, Akikusa B, Takazawa H, Okabayashi A. A histopathologic study of early hepatocellular carcinoma. Cancer 1983;52:687–692.
9. Kojiro M, Sugihara S, Nakashima O. Pathomorphologic characteristics of early hepatocellular carcinoma. In: Okuda K, Tobe T, Kitagawa T (eds) Early Detection and Treatment of Liver Cancer. Tokyo: Japan Scientific Societies Press, 1991:29–33.
10. Kiyomatsu K. Pathomorphologic study on early hepatocellular carcinoma-A study of fatty change. Acta Hepatol Jpn 1997;30:974–979. (in Japanese.)
11. Kenmochi K, Sugihara S, Kojiro M. Relationship of histologic grade of hepatocellular carcinoma (HCC) to tumor size, and demonstration of tumor cells of multiple different grades in a single small HCC. Liver 1987;7:18–26.
12. Yano H, Iemura A, Fukuda K, Mizoguchi A, Haramaki M, Kojiro M. Establishment of two distinct human hepatocellular carcinoma cell lines from a single nodule showing clonal dedifferentiation of cancer cells. Hepatology 1993;18:320–327.

Progress in Hepatology, Volume 3.
Hepatocellular Carcinoma.
M. Yamanaka, G. Toda and T. Tanaka, editors.

Genomic changes and development of hepatocellular carcinoma

Shuichi Kaneko, Rieko Saeki and Kenichi Kobayashi
First Department of Internal Medicine, Kanazawa University School of Medicine, Kanazawa, Japan

Abstract. Recent studies support the idea that accumulation of genetic changes underlie the cancer development, and multistep process is well-illustrated by colorectal cancer. Genomic changes during hepatocellular carcinoma (HCC) development show small HCCs consisted of well-differentiated cancer cells, large HCCs consisted of heterogeneous population of less-differentiated cells, and metastatic tumors were studied using restriction landmark genomic scanning method (RLGS). Two small HCCs consisted of well-differentiated cells and four large HCCs with partitions by fibrous septa in a single nodule were analyzed. Intra-tumoral genetic heterogeneity was not found in the two small HCCs but only in the four HCCs. The number of genomic changes in HCCs ranging 7 to 95 mm in diameter were analyzed. Less than 11 spots in RLGS profile were different in small size of HCC, whereas more than 35 spots were different in large size of HCC, indicating that the number of genetic changes increase with the tumor size. Genomic changes among two nodules in a liver of five patients were studied to differentiate clonal origin of the nodules. Three of the five patients demonstrated that the two nodules were genetically apart; and the two nodules of the remaining two patients were similar, indicating unifocal intra-hepatic metastasis. Thus, relationship between the number of genetic changes and the development of HCC was shown in this study.

Keywords: cancer, gene, genomic heterogeneity, intrahepatic metastasis, metastasis, mutation, restriction landmark genomic scanning (RLGS).

Introduction

Carcinogenesis is now considered a highly complicated process in which accumulative mutations in oncogenes and tumor suppressor genes are required for transformation of a normal cell to a malignant cell. Any one of several mechanisms such as point mutation, translocation, amplification, deletion, or loss of chromosomes can activate oncogenes or inactivate tumor suppressor genes and allow a cell to escape from normal control of growth. Successive mutations allow the cell to obtain more malignant phenotypes such as rapid growth and metastasis [1—3]. Multiple genomic mutations have been reported in hepatocellular carcinomas (HCCs) such as allelic losses [4—6] and p53 gene mutation [7—10]. The mutations, however, have been detected only in relatively advanced large HCC, and other genomic mutations are considered to occur during cancer development.

Recent advances in diagnostic modalities have facilitated the detection of HCCs as small as 0.5 cm in diameter of HCC. Small HCC less than 1.5 cm in

Address for correspondence: Shuichi Kaneko, First Department of Internal Medicine, Kanazawa University School of Medicine, Takara-Machi 13-1, Kanazawa 920, Japan. Tel.: +81-762-62-8151. Fax: +81-762-34-4250. E-mail: skaneko@med.kanazawa-u.ac.jp diameter usually shows homogeneous histological appearance consisting of well-differentiated cancer cells, and larger HCC shows moderately or poorly differentiated cancer cells. When an HCC nodule contains another discrete nodule inside the nodule, this is called a "nodule-in-nodule" appearance, consisting of more malignant cancer cells [11,12]. These histological findings suggest that a cancer cell clonally expands to a small tumor, a more malignant cancer cell inside the tumor arises causing rapid growing cancer cells to dominate the tumor. From recent studies in colorectal cancers, these changes correlate with multiple genetic mutations [13]. However, the identification of responsible genes to the histological changes and the number of genetic mutations have not been systematically studied in HCC.

Restriction landmark genomic scanning (RLGS), a two-dimensional DNA electrophoresis method, is suited to detect genomic changes in chromosomal DNA [14—17]. In RLGS, end-labeled restriction enzyme sites are used as landmarks in a gel so that 2,000—3,000 landmarks distributed throughout the genome can be surveyed in one procedure. We performed RLGS and demonstrated the relationship between histological difference and genetic heterogeneity in HCCs.

Materials and Methods

HCC samples

All HCC nodules were previously untreated and surgically removed from patients. A small section was taken from HCC nodule and from the noncancerous region. In the cases showing several partitions inside the tumor, samples (2—3 mm square) were taken from two different parts (A,B). A fraction of the samples was fixed in neutral 10% formaldehyde for histological examinations, and the remainders were immediately frozen and stored at $-80°C$ until there was an isolation of DNA. High-molecular weight DNA was carefully extracted from each sample by digestion with proteinase K followed by phenol/chloroform extraction. The fixed samples were embedded in paraffin, sliced and stained with hematoxylin and eosin. The histological typing was done according to the World Health Organization criteria [18]. The degree of tumor differentiation was estimated according to Edmondson and Steiner [19].

RLGS

RLGS analysis was performed as described previously [14,15]. High molecular weight DNA (10 μg) was prepared and subjected to blocking reaction, digested with Not I, end-labeled with [^{32}P]deoxycytidine 5′-triphosphate and [^{32}P]deoxyguanosine 5′-triphosphate (6,000 Ci/mmol, NEN, Boston, USA), and then digested with EcoR V for size fractionation. After the first dimensional gel electrophoresis, the sample was digested in situ with Hinf I, and electrophoresed for the second dimension. After electrophoresis and autoradiography, radioactivity of spots was measured using a Bio-image analyzer BAS 2000 (Fuji Film, Kanagawa, Japan).

The RLGS offers a sensitivity that cannot only detect appearance of new spots or disappearance of an old spot, but also distinguish diploid from haploid genomes, since each spot that originates from a diploid region of the genome should show identical radioactivity, if both paternal and maternal chromosomal DNAs are equally cleaved by Not I, and labeled. Then, the intensity of a spot originating from a haploid genome should be a half of that of diploid genome.

About 2,000 spots were obtained by RLGS. In each case, the RLGS profile of HCC sample was first compared with that of noncancerous sample. Spots that were different in intensity were recorded. All changes including appearance, disappearance and different intensity in each spot were counted as different spots indicating genomic heterogeneity of the sample.

Results and Discussion

Intra-tumoral genomic heterogeneity

A large body of evidence supports the idea that accumulated genetic changes underlie the development of cancer, and multistep process is well illustrated by colorectal cancers [13]. As one of the unique features of HCC development, histological heterogeneity existing in a single tumor nodule is known. Histological examination of advanced HCC demonstrates that there are several compartments in a single tumor nodule. When an HCC tumor contains another discrete nodule, this is called a "nodule-in-nodule" appearance [11,12]. It is interesting to know whether the genetic changes exist in a single HCC nodule. We performed RLGS in two distinct parts of four advanced HCCs along with two different regions of two small and homogeneous HCCs (Table 1). HCCs from cases 1—4 were over 20 mm in diameter. The tumor nodule of the four was divided into several parts by fibrous septa. HCCs from cases 5 and 6 were less than 15 mm in diameter and demonstrated homogeneous surface. In cases 1—4 showing several partitions inside the tumor, three samples (2—3 mm square) were taken from two different parts (A,B) as well as from the noncancerous region (C). Similar sections were

Table 1. Genomic changes in a single HCC nodule. Four HCCs (cases 1—4) have partitions by fibrous septa, and two different parts (A,B) were analyzed with the nontumour part (C). Two HCCs (cases 5—6) have histologically homogenous appearance, and two distant parts were similarly analyzed. The number of different spots (A and C, B and C) and the number of commonly differerent spots (B and C) were shown.

Case	1		2		3		4		5		6	
Tumor size (mm)	45		45		25		20		7		10	
Sample	1A	1B	2A	2B	3A	3B	4A	4B	5A	5B	6A	6B
Edmondson-Steiner grade	II	II	II	II	II	II	III	III	I	I	I	I

also obtained from two independent regions (A,B) of a tumor from the cases 5 and 6, and from the nontumorous region (C).

In case 1, 55 spots were different in intensity between A and C, and 57 spots between B and C. Among these spots, 54 spots were common between A and B. Thirty-five of them were intensified, and 19 were dwindled in the cancer. In case 2, 68 spots were different in intensity between A and C, and 62 spots between B and C. Among these spots, 56 spots were common between A and B. Thirty-six of them were intensified and 20 were dwindled in cancer. In case 3, 57 spots were different in intensity between A and C, and 59 spots were between B and C. Among these spots, 52 spots were common between A and B. Forty-one of them were intensified, and 11 were dwindled in cancer. In case 4, 39 spots were different in intensity between A and C, and 40 spots between B and C. Among these spots, 37 spots were common between A and B. Thirty-one of them were intensified, and 6 were dwindled in cancer. Thus, DNAs from cancerous regions A and B share many chromosomal changes compared with noncancerous region C. Similar analyses were done with two HCCs (cases 5 and 6). In case 5, regions A and B obtained from different regions of a tumor, showed indistinguishable profiles, although six spots were different between A or B and C. In case 6, three spots were different between A or B and C, and again, A and B were arbitrarily chosen from the different regions of a tumor, showed identical profiles. Thus, there were no clonal differences in regions A and B of cases 5 and 6.

Intra-tumoral heterogeneity in the chromosomal DNA was clearly demonstrated with the four tumors that demonstrated the inside partitions. In contrast, two small HCCs that looked homogeneous did not show such chromosomal heterogeneity. Contribution of "nodule-in-nodule" formation or the inside partition to cancer progression is not known, but tumors around 2 cm or more in diameter often show such appearances that have shown to have acquired independent mutations. In addition, the "nodule-in-nodule" region tends to consist of less-differentiated cells surrounded by more-differentiated cells as the tumor size increases. Thus, it has been hypothesized that genetic alterations occur inside the more-differentiated tumor, the altered cell forms a less-differentiated nodule inside the tumor, resulting in "nodule-in-nodule" or the partition formation, within which poorly differentiated cells appear and become dominant when they bear an advanced HCC.

Tumor size and genomic heterogeneity

Ten HCC samples ranging 7 to 95 mm in diameter were analyzed by RLGS to find out whether the number of genetic changes correlate with the tumor size or histological malignancy (Table 2). Four samples smaller than 20 mm in diameter consisted of well-differentiated cancer cells, and six samples larger than 36 mm consisted of moderately or poorly differentiated cancer cells. Three to 58 among about 2,000 spots in RLGS were different between HCC and the corresponding

Table 2. Tumor size and genomic changes. Ten HCC samples were analyzed by RLGS, and the profile was compared with that from the corresponding nontumorous liver. The number of the different spots was shown.

Case	1	2	3	4	5	6	7	8	9	10
Tumor size (mm)	7	8	15	20	36	40	40	40	80	95
No. of different spots	8	11	3	9	35	55	58	54	50	41

nontumorous liver. Less than 11 spots were different in small size of HCC (cases 1–4), whereas more than 35 spots were different in large size of HCC (cases 5–10). Thus, genomic heterogeneity between HCC and the corresponding nontumorous liver increased with the tumor size and/or differentiation of cancer cells. These findings indicate that genomic mutations accumulate with HCC expansion or cellular differentiation, and the mutation or combination of the mutations may be responsible for the histological changes.

Intrahepatic metastasis and genomic heterogeneity

Genomic changes between the two nodules in a liver were studied to analyze whether or not the nodules come from the same clonal origin. Two different HCC nodules in a liver were obtained from five patients; the larger one was named T1, and the other one T2 (Table 3). Case 1 had two HCCs in the liver. T1 was 4 cm in diameter and moderately differentiated, T2 was small (1.0 cm) and consisted of highly well-differentiated cells. Seven spots in T1 were different from spots in the nontumorous part of the liver, and 17 in T2. There was only one common spot difference in T1 and T2. Case 2 had two small HCCs. T1 was 1.5 cm in diameter and moderately differentiated, T2 was 0.7 cm and well differentiated. Similarly, 12 spots in T1 were different, six in T2, and one spot was commonly different from those in the nontumorous liver. Case 3 had two large HCCs. T1 consisted of moderately differentiated cells with trabecular pattern, T2 had poorly differentiated cells with scirrhous pattern. Case 4 had three large HCC nodules with portal vein tumor thrombus. Two nodules in the right lobe were analyzed. Both of these tumors demonstrated moderately differentiated HCC with trabecular pattern. Twenty-seven spots in T1 were different, eight in T2, but all the eight different spots were similarly found in T1 indicating all the

Table 3. Genomic changes and intra-hepatic nodules. Two HCC nodules in a liver of five patients were analyzed by RLGS. The larger nodule was named T1 and the smaller T2.

Case	1		2		3		4		5	
Nodule	T1	T2	T1	T2	T1	T2	T1	T2	T1	T2
Tumor size (mm)	40	10	15	7	40	30	100	40	50	20
Edmondson-Steiner grade	II	II	III	I	II	IV	II	II	II	III
No. of different spots	7	17	12	6	60	17	27	8	50	46
No. of commonly different spots	1		1		2		8		42	

genomic changes found in T2 also present in T1. Case 5 had a large HCC (T1 5.0 cm) and a lot of surrounding small nodules. One of these small nodules was analyzed (T2). Both T1 and T2 demonstrated moderately differentiated HCC with trabecular pattern. Fifty spots in T1 were different, 46 in T2, and similarly to case 4, 42 of the 46 were commonly found in T1. These findings suggest that the two nodules in cases 1 to 3 were genetically distant compared with the two nodules found in cases 4 and 5, which share many genetic heterogeneity.

Thus, RLGS demonstrated genomic heterogeneity among nodules in a liver, and may be useful in understanding the clonal origin and differentiate multifocal tumor development from unifocal intra-hepatic metastasis. The mechanism for genomic heterogeneity in RLGS has been studied. Methylation or demethylation, to which the restriction enzyme Not I used for the end-labeling of landmarks is sensitive, or amplification, deletion or loss of heterozygosity are the most likely cancers [14,15]. Clarification of responsible mutations for RLGS change should be useful for understanding the relation between the gene and tumor progression. Regardless of the mechanism of the genetic changes in RLGS, this study clearly demonstrates that genomic heterogeneity is less common in the small more-differentiated cancer, genomic changes occur even in a single HCC nodule, and increase during the tumor expansion and metastasis.

References

1. Fearon ER, Vogelstein B. A genetic model for colorectal tumorigenesis. Cell 1990;61:759–767.
2. Hamilton SR. Molecular genetics of colorectal carcinoma. Cancer 1992;70:1216–1221.
3. Vogelstein B, Kinzler KW. The multistep nature of cancer. Trend Genet 1993;9:138–141.
4. Fujimori M, Tokino T, Hino O, Kitagawa T, Imamura T, Okamoto E, Mitsunobu M et al. Allelotype study of primary hepatocellular carcinoma. Cancer Res 1991;51:89–93.
5. Walker GJ, Hayward NK, Falvey S, Cooksley WGE. Loss of somatic heterozygosity in hepatocellular carcinoma. Cancer Res 1991;51:4367–4370.
6. Takahashi K, Kudo J, Ishibashi H, Hirata Y, Niho Y. Frequent loss of heterozygosity on chromosome 22 in hepatocellular carcinoma. Hepatology 1993;17:794–799.
7. Bressac B, Galvin KM, Liang TJ, Isselbacher KJ, Wands JR. Abnormal structure and expression of p53 gene in human hepatocellular carcinoma. Proc Natl Acad Sci USA 1990;87:1973–1977.
8. Hsu IC, Metcalf RA, Sun T, Welsh JA, Wang NJ, Harris CC. Mutation hot spot in the p53 gene in human hepatocellular carcinomas. Nature 1991;350:427–428.
9. Murakami Y, Hayashi K, Sekiya T. Detection of aberrations of the p53 alleles and the gene transcript in human tumor cell lines by single-strand conformation polymorphism analysis. Cancer Res 1991;51:3356–3361.
10. Oda T, Tsuda H, Scarpa A, Sakamoto M, Hirohashi S. p53 gene mutation spectrum in hepatocellular carcinoma. Cancer Res 1992;52:6358–6364.
11. Popper H. Pathological aspects of cirrhosis. A review. Am J Pathol 1977;87:228–264.
12. Arakawa M, Kage M, Sugihara S, Nakashima T, Suenaga M, Okuda K. Emergence of malignant lesions within an adenomatous hyperplastic nodule in a cirrhotic liver. Observations in five cases. Gastroenterology 1986;91:198–208.
13. Kenneth WK, Vogelstein B. Lessons from hereditary colorectal cancer. Cell 1996;87:159–170.
14. Hatada I, Hayashizaki Y, Hirotsune S, Komatsubara H, Mukai T. A genomic scanning method for higher organisms using restriction sites as landmarks. Proc Natl Acad Sci USA 1991;88:9523–9527.

15. Hirotsune S, Hatada I, Komatsubara H, Nagai H, Kuma K, Kobayakawa K, Kawara T et al. New approach for detection of amplification in cancer DNA using restriction landmark genomic scanning. Cancer Res 1992;52:3642–3647.
16. Nagai H, Hirotsune S, Komatsubara H, Hatada I, Mukai T, Hayashizaki Y, Matsubara K. Genomic analysis of human hepatocellular carcinomas using restriction landmark genomic scanning. Cancer Detec Prev 1993;17:399–404.
17. Nagai H, Ponglikitmongkol M, Mita E, Ohmachi Y, Yoshikawa H, Saeki R, Yumoto Y, Nakanishi T, Matsubara, K. Aberration of genomic DNA in association with human hepatocellular carcinomas detected by 2-D analysis. Cancer Res 1994;54:1545–1550.
18. WHO histological typing of tumours of the liver, biliary tract and pancreas. Second edn. Springer-Verlag, 1994.
19. Edmondson HA, Steiner PE. Primary carcinoma of the liver: a study of 100 cases among 48,900 necropsies. Cancer 1954;7:462–503.

©1997 Elsevier Science B.V. All rights reserved.
Progress in Hepatology, Volume 3.
Hepatocellular Carcinoma.
M. Yamanaka, G. Toda and T. Tanaka, editors.

Color Doppler energy as a diagnostic modality for small hepatocellular carcinoma

Akiko Saito
Department of Gastroenterology, Tokyo Women's Medical College, Tokyo, Japan

Abstract. Color Doppler energy (CDE) offers a marked improvement in sensitivity over existing color Doppler systems. This report describes the use of this system in diagnosing small hepatocellular carcinoma (HCC). CDE was used in the clinical investigation of 32 nodules, 2 cm or less in diameter, in 31 HCC cases. Findings were compared with those obtained by ordinary color Doppler imaging (CDI), angioechography and histopathological examination. The apparatus was an Acuson 128XP/10 (ART) with 4- and 5-MHz transducers. Both CDI and CDE showed pulsatile flow but with marked differences in sensitivity. Flow was intermittent or spotty with CDI, while mainly a continuous branched pattern was visualized with CDE. CDE showed pulsatile flow in 13 of the 16 nodules (81.3%) in which angioechography showed positive enhancement. In all seven nodules in which angioechography showed negative or nonenhancement, no pulsatile flow was seen on CDE. Twelve of 14 nodules with moderate or poor differentiation histopathologically showed continuous pulsatile flow on CDE. Among 18 well-differentiated HCCs, no pulsatile flow was seen in 14, intermittent pulsatile flow in three and spotty flow in one.

Thus, CDE images correlated well with angioechographic and histopathological findings. CDE is an effective and noninvasive means of determining the feeding artery and is useful for diagnosing small HCC.

Keywords: angioechography, color Doppler ultrasonography, hemodynamics, liver tumor, small hepatocellular carcinoma, ultrasonography.

Introduction

The Doppler system is widely used to examine the hemodynamic features of the liver. To date, however, the sensitivity of this modality has been insufficient for tumor diagnosis.

A new mode of Doppler ultrasonography, color Doppler energy (CDE), was recently developed [1]. The innovative feature of this system is based on increased sensitivity to flow, with little angle dependence and no aliasing. This is because color flow on CDE displays the integrated power of the Doppler signal instead of its mean Doppler frequency shift.

As we already reported, CDE offers markedly enhanced sensitivity over existing color Doppler imaging (CDI) and allows substantial improvement in the diagnosis of hepatocellular carcinoma (HCC) [2].

Address for correspondence: Akiko Saito MD, Institute of Gastroenterology, Tokyo Women's Medical College, 8-1 Kawada-cho, Shinjuku-ku, Tokyo 162, Japan. Tel.: +81-3-3353-8111. Fax: +81-3-5269-7435.

The use of this system, in the diagnosis of 31 cases of small HCC, is described in this paper.

Patients and Methods

Thirty-two nodules in 31 consecutive HCC cases detected from 1994 through 1995 were investigated. These cases were selected among patients undergoing CDE in whom nodule size was shown to be 2 cm or less. The nodules were histopathologically confirmed with 25 resected specimens and seven needle biopsies. CDE findings of the 32 nodules were compared with those of CDI, angioechography and histopathological differentiation.

Angioechography is a simple form of enhanced ultrasonography employing direct injection of a small amount of carbon dioxide gas (1—5 ml) via the proper hepatic artery [3]. Angioechography of the tumor can be divided into three patterns (Fig. 1).

The apparatus used was an Acuson 128XP/10 (ART) color Doppler ultrasound (Acuson Corp., Mountain View, CA, USA) equipped with 4-MHz (vector type) and 5-MHz (curved array) transducers.

Results

Comparison of CDI and CDE findings (Table 1)

CDI showed pulsatile flow in 13 of 32 nodules. CDE also showed pulsatile flow in 16 nodules, but with greater sensitivity. With CDI, flow was intermittent in nine and spotty in four, while on CDE a continuous branched pattern was visual-

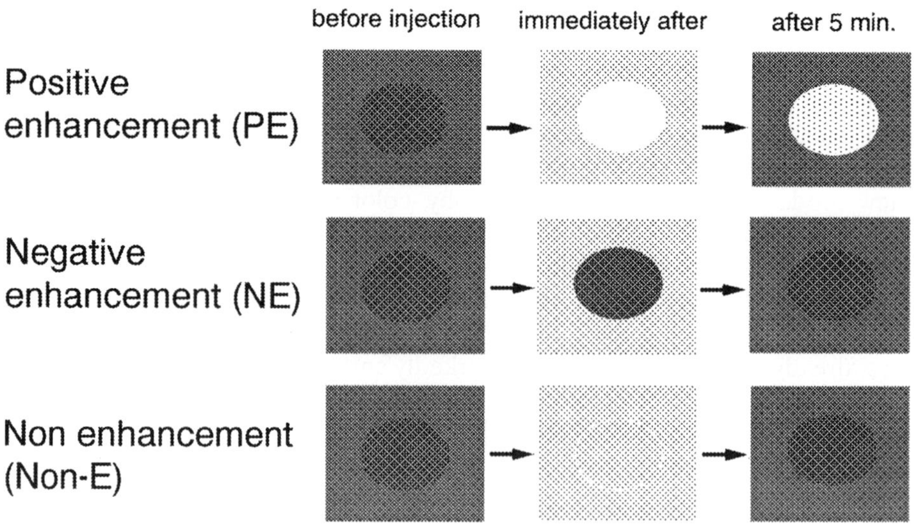

Fig. 1. Angioechographic patterns.

Table 1. Comparison of CDI and CDE findings.

CDI	CDE			
	Continuous pulsatile flow	Intermittent pulsatile flow	Spotty pulsatile flow	(−)
Intermittent (n = 9)	8	1		
Spotty (n = 4)	3	1		
(−) (n = 19)	1	1	1	16

ized in 12 nodules, an intermittent pattern in three and a spotty pattern in only one.

Comparison of angioechographic and CDE findings (Table 2)

CDE showed continuous pulsatile flow in 12 and spotty flow in one of the 16 positively enhanced nodules (PE). In the remaining three nodules, a CDE image could not be obtained due to interruption by the pulsatile movement of the intestine in one and observational difficulty, i.e., a location in the dome of right hepatic lobe, in two. In the seven nodules with a small area of positive enhancement surrounded by negative enhancement (PE+NE), CDE showed intermittent pulsatile flow. Moreover, in the seven nodules which showed negative (NE) or non-enhancement (Non-E), CDE images confirmed the absence of pulsatile flow.

Comparison of pathological and CDE findings (Table 3)

Twelve of 14 nodules with moderate or poor differentiation histopathologically showed continuous pulsatile flow on CDE. Among 18 well-differentiated HCC, 14 showed no pulsatile flow, while in three nodules flow was intermittent pulsatile and in one spotty.

Case presentation (Fig. 2)

A typical example of hypervasculer HCC. Conventional ultrasonography revealed an isoechoic nodule with a hypoechoic rim in segment 5 (Fig. 2c,left). CDI

Table 2. Comparison of angiographic and CDE findings.

Angioecho	CDE			
	Continuous pulsatile flow	Intermittent pulsatile flow	Spotty pulsatile flow	(−)
PE (n = 16)	12		1	3
NE + PE (n = 7)		3		4
NE (n = 6)				6
Non-E − NE (n = 1)				1

Table 3. Comparison of histopathological and CDE findings.

Differentiation of HCC	CDE			
	Continuous pulsatile flow	Intermittent pulsatile flow	Spotty pulsatile flow	(−)
Moderate to poor (n = 14)	12			2
Well (n = 18)		3	1	14

showed indistinct intermittent blood flow (Fig. 2a). In contrast, CDE depicted clear pulsatile flow into the nodule as an uninterrupted image (Fig. 2b). On angioechography, the nodule appeared as positive enhancement (Fig. 2c,right). The resected specimen showed an encapsulated, 1.3-cm nodule which was histopathologically confirmed to be a moderately differentiated HCC.

Discussion

CDE, or Power Doppler as it is generally known, was initially introduced in the cardiac field, and is now used in the gastroenterological, renal and other fields [4–6].

Employing this modality in hypervascular small HCC allows uninterrupted pulsatile imaging, comparable to that achieved with angiography or angioechography, of the blood flow in vessels entering the tumor. CDE is superior, however, in that clear, real-time flow is depicted noninvasively.

Even in hypervascular nodules as small as 9 mm, CDE facilitated detection of the feeding artery under appropriate ultrasonographic conditions. Otherwise, images could not be obtained in some cases due to observational difficulty or interference from the pulsatile movement of the intestine, heart and so on.

CDE also offers advantages in the detection of hypovascular HCC. Currently, the easiest and most sensitive way to demonstrate hypovascular HCC is by angioechography. Hypovascular nodules as visualized by this modality appear as negative enhancement (NE). CDE may depict the lack of an intra-tumor feeding artery in such cases.

Based on the results obtained in these cases, CDE provides clear differentiation of hypo- from hypervascular nodules. Distinguishing between such lesions is anticipated to minimize the utilization of needle biopsy in unsuitable hypervascular cases, i.e., moderately or poorly differentiated HCC, a procedure which may result in the dissemination of malignant cells. In these cases, angiography or angioechography may be performed after CDE for confirmation of the diagnosis. Furthermore, with CDE, angiography is unnecessary in hypovascular cases, making it possible to proceed directly to biopsy in order to distinguish well-differentiated HCC from a large regenerated nodule.

In summary, CDE images showed excellent correlations with angioechographic and histopathological findings. CDE is an effective and noninvasive means of

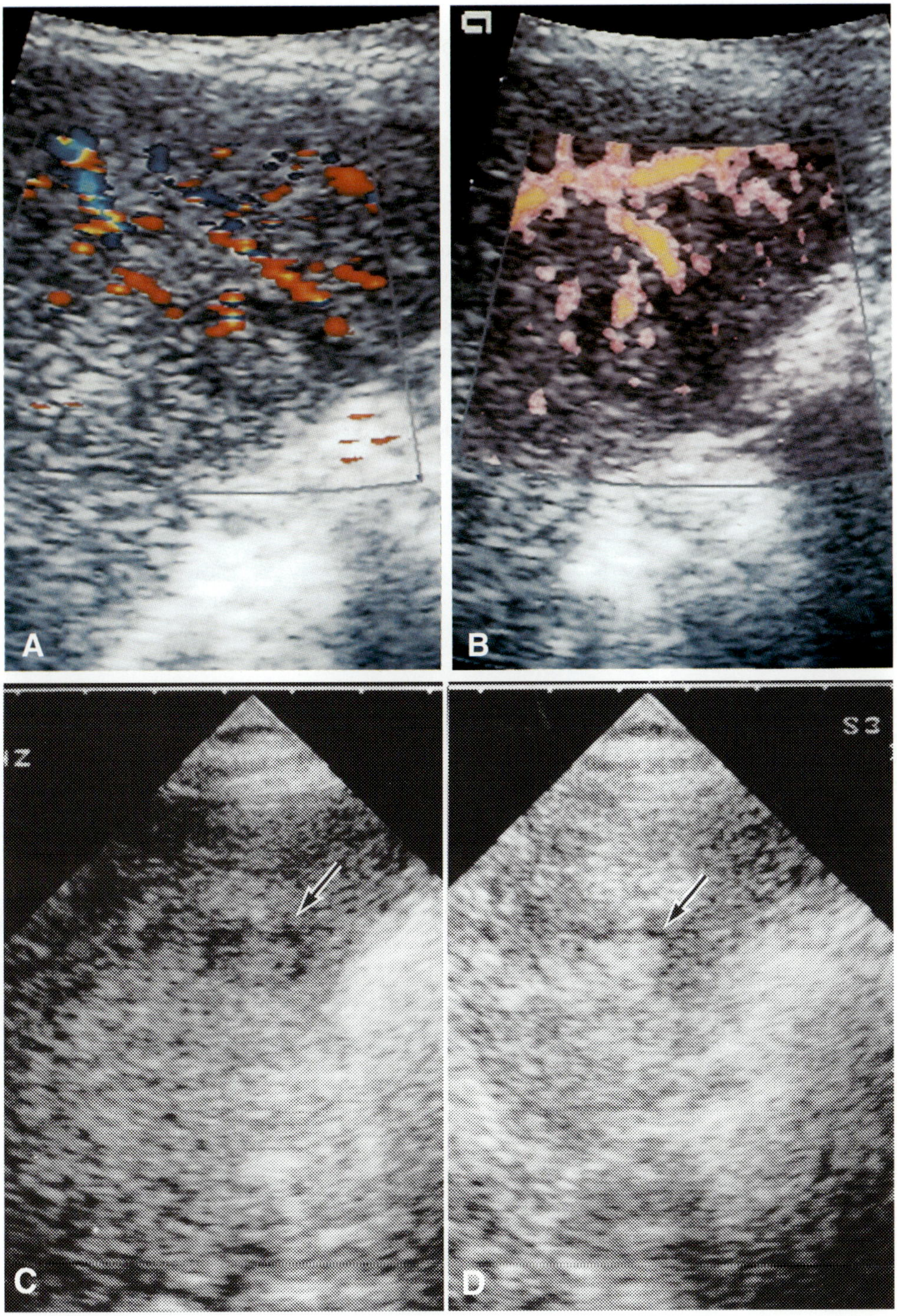

Fig. 2. A case of hypervascular HCC. **A**: CDI, **B**: CDE, **C**: angioechography before CO_2 injection, **D**: angioechography immediately after injection.

assessing the hemodynamics of small nodules and is useful for diagnosing small HCC.

References

1. Rubin JM, Adler RS. Power Doppler expands standard color Doppler capability. Diagnost Imag 1993;15(12):66–69.
2. Saito A, Sugimoto C, Niinami C et al. Use of color Doppler energy in the diagnosis of small hepatocellular carcinoma. International Hepatology Communications 1995;4:160–164.
3. Saito A, Takasaki T, Nakagawa M et al. Angio-echo method under intravascular carbon dioxide gas injection for liver tumor. Kan-Tan-Sui 1987;15(6):1129–1132. (in Japanese)
4. Newman NS, Adler RS, Bude RO et al. Detection of soft tissue hyperemia: value of power Doppler sonography. AJR 1994;163:385–389.
5. Rubin JM, Bude RO, Carson PL et al. Power Doppler US: A potentially useful alternative to mean frequency-based Color Doppler US. Radiology 1994;190:853–856.
6. Bude RO, Rubin JM, Adler RS. Power versus conventional color Doppler sonography: comparison in the depiction of normal intrarenal vasculature. Radiology 1994;192:777–780.

Progress in Hepatology, Volume 3.
Hepatocellular Carcinoma.
M. Yamanaka, G. Toda and T. Tanaka, editors.

Prospective study of chemoprevention of hepatocellular carcinoma with a Chinese herbal medicine

Hiroko Oka[1] and Sukeo Yamamoto[2]
[1]Department of Gastroenterology, Osaka City General Hospital, Osaka; and [2]The Third Department of Internal Medicine, Osaka City University Medical School, Osaka, Japan

Abstract. A prospective, randomized, nonblind controlled study was performed to evaluate the preventive effect of Sho-saiko-to (TJ-9) on hepatocellular carcinoma (HCC) development. TJ-9 is a Chinese herbal medicine that contains crude extracts of seven herbs. Two hundred and sixty patients with cirrhosis were randomly assigned to two groups matched for their backgrounds. The patients in the trial group were given TJ-9 at a daily dose of 7.5 g in addition to the conventional drugs given to the control group. The patients were prospectively monitored for 60 months and the cumulative incidence of HCC and the survival rate in the two groups were calculated.

The cumulative incidence curve for 5 years of the trial group was lower than that of the control group. For the patients without HBs antigen, the difference was significant. The survival curve for 5 years of the trial group was higher than that of the control group. For the patients without HBs antigen, the difference was significant.

TJ-9 helped to prevent the development of HCC in patients with cirrhosis, particularly in patients without HBs antigen.

Keywords: Chinese herbal medicine, hepatoma, prevention and control, Sho-saiko-to.

Introduction

Hepatocellular carcinoma (HCC) is one of the most common cancers in the world, with an estimated 500,000 to 1 million new cases diagnosed yearly. More than 80% of patients with HCC have underlying cirrhosis [1], and the yearly incidence of HCC being diagnosed in cirrhotic patients was 7% in studies in Japan [2,3]. Recently, it became possible to detect HCC in the early stage by ultrasonography, computed tomography and the assay of α-fetoprotein (AFP). HCC is suitable for investigation of the efficacy of potential chemopreventive drugs. Firstly, patients with cirrhosis are at high risk for HCC; and secondly, the follow-up period before HCC can be detected is short. We reported the study of a prospective randomized nonblind controlled trial undertaken in an evaluation of the chemopreventive effect of a Chinese herbal medicine, Sho-saiko-to (TJ-9) [4], here we summarized the content of the study.

Address for correspondence: Hiroko Oka MD, Department of Gastroenterology, Osaka City General Hospital, 2-53 Miyakojima-hondori, Miyakojima-ku, Osaka 534, Japan.

Patients and Methods

Patients

Two hundred and sixty outpatients with cirrhosis were monitored for 60 months beginning June, 1985, at the Third Department of Internal Medicine, Osaka City University Medical School and affiliated hospitals. The patients were 164 men and 96 women, with a mean age of 58 years (range, 31–84 years). On entry into the study, the patients were examined by ultrasonography to rule out the presence of HCC. The patients all had AFP levels below 200 ng/ml 3 months or less before entry. Thirty-seven patients had hepatitis B surface antigen (HBsAg) and 223 patients had not. Tests for anti-C100-3 antibodies gave positive results for 76 of the 94 patients whose sera were tested.

Patients were classified by age, sex, presence of HBsAg and liver dysfunction score, which was based on the levels of serum albumin, bilirubin and cholinesterase (Table 1). The score was significantly related to the incidence of HCC in our previous study [5]. Patients of the same sex, age, liver dysfunction score, and presence of HBsAg were classified as subgroups. In the same subgroup, patients were randomly assigned to the control group or the trial group. The patients in the control group received conventional medicine only; those in the trial group were given TJ-9 at the daily dose of 7.5 g orally in addition to the conventional medicine. All patients started conventional therapy, and when a matched patient became available, randomization to treatment took place. Informed consent was obtained from the patients before they entered the study. All patients were prospectively followed up by monitoring of the serum level of AFP every 2 months and by ultrasonography scanning every 3 months. The mean length and the standard deviation of the follow-up period was 38.4 ± 22.3 months (median, 41 months).

Table 2 shows the background of the patients at entry into the study. There was no significant difference in any test between the two groups.

Methods

Ultrasonography was done with convex-array real-time scanners. HCC was diagnosed from the finding of typical hypervascular characteristics by angiography in addition to generally accepted features of HCC seen by computed tomography

Table 1. Liver dysfunction score.

Score	Serum bilirubin (mg/dl)	Serum albumin (g/dl)	Serum cholinesterase (pH change)
0	< 1.5	> 4.0	> 0.60
1	1.5–3.0	3.0–4.0	0.40–0.60
2	> 3.0	< 3.0	< 0.40

Table 2. Profiles and laboratory data of patients at the time of entry into the study.

Data	Trial group	Control group
Patient characteristics		
Sex (M/F)	82:48	82:48
Age (yr)	58 ± 9	59 ± 9
HBsAg detected	16/130	21/130
History of blood transfusion	24/130	30/130
History of heavy drinking	23/130	34/130
Laboratory data		
AFP	29.2 ± 48.6	23.1 ± 35.0
AST	104.4 ± 61.6	91.8 ± 60.2
ALT	130.3 ± 103.5	107.4 ± 86.9
γ-GTP	46.4 ± 27.7	45.0 ± 51.2
Cholinesterase	0.50 ± 0.18	0.48 ± 0.18
Total bilirubin	1.24 ± 0.63	1.26 ± 0.77
Albumin	3.6 ± 0.5	3.5 ± 0.6
Liver dysfunction score	2.0 ± 1.5	1.9 ± 1.4

and ultrasonography. When ultrasonography findings suggested the presence of HCC but angiography did not show typical images of HCC, a biopsy specimen was obtained under ultrasonography guidance.

Evaluation of chemoprevention effects

The chemopreventive effect of TJ-9 was evaluated by the cumulative incidence of HCC and survival rates. Patients in whom HCC was detected within 6 months after entry were excluded to rule out patients who had a large number of HCC cells but not enough to be detectable at the time of entry into the study.

Statistical analysis

The cumulative incidence of HCC was computed by the method of Gaynor et al. [6]. The differences between the cumulative incidence were analyzed by the test proposed by Gray [7], because some patients died without HCC. For comparison of the survival between the two treatment arms, the log rank test was used.

Results

Cumulative incidence of HCC

HCC was found in 63 of the 260 patients during the follow-up period. Seven patients were found to have HCC within 6 months from the entry and were excluded. Forty-seven of the patients not found to have HCC died 6–60 months after entering the study. The most common causes of death were liver failure and variceal bleeding. One hundred and ninety-one patients survived until the end of the follow-up period. TJ-9 had no undesired side effects.

Figure 1 shows the curves of the cumulative incidence of HCC in the treated and control groups during the trial. There were 23 (23%) patients with HCC in the trial group and 33 (34%) patients with HCC in the control group. The incidence of HCC was lower in the trial group ($p = 0.071$).

At the time of entry by patients not later excluded, 184 patients had AFP levels below 20 ng/ml. Among the remaining 69 patients who had AFP levels between 20 and 199 and ng/ml, only 11 patients had AFP levels $\geqslant 100$ ng/ml. Figure 2 shows the cumulative incidence of HCC during the 5-year follow-up study in the 184 patients who had AFP levels < 20 ng/ml at entry. The incidence of HCC was 21% (15 cases) in the trial group and 28% (19 cases) in the control group ($p = 0.335$). Figure 3 shows the cumulative incidence of HCC in the 69 patients who had AFP levels of > 20 ng/ml but below 200 ng/ml. The incidence of HCC was 27% (8 cases) in the trial group and 50% (14 cases) in the control group ($p = 0.062$).

Figure 4 shows the cumulative incidence of HCC in the patients without HBsAg. The incidence was significantly lower in the trial group (22%) than in the control group (39%) ($p = 0.024$).

Survival rate

Figure 5 shows the cumulative survival curves of the patients with cirrhosis (some with HCC) in the two groups. The survival curve was higher for the trial group

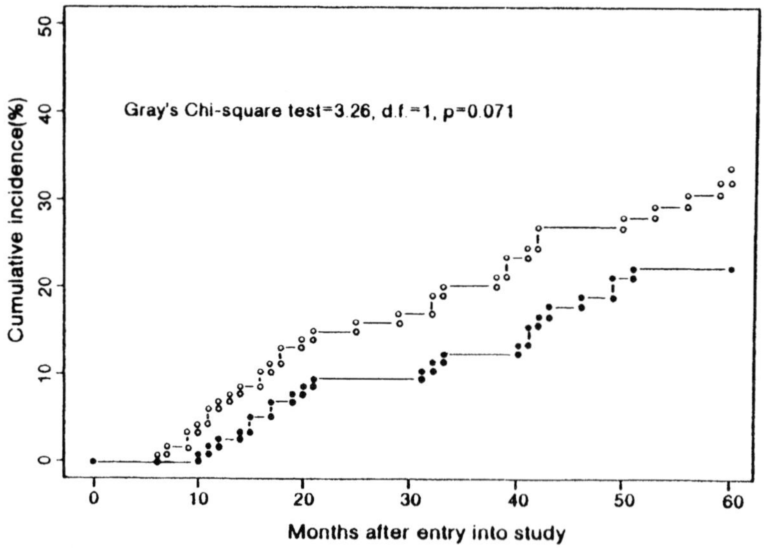

Fig. 1. Cumulative incidence of HCC detected 6 months or more after entry into the study. ●: trial group (n = 127); ○: control group (n = 126).

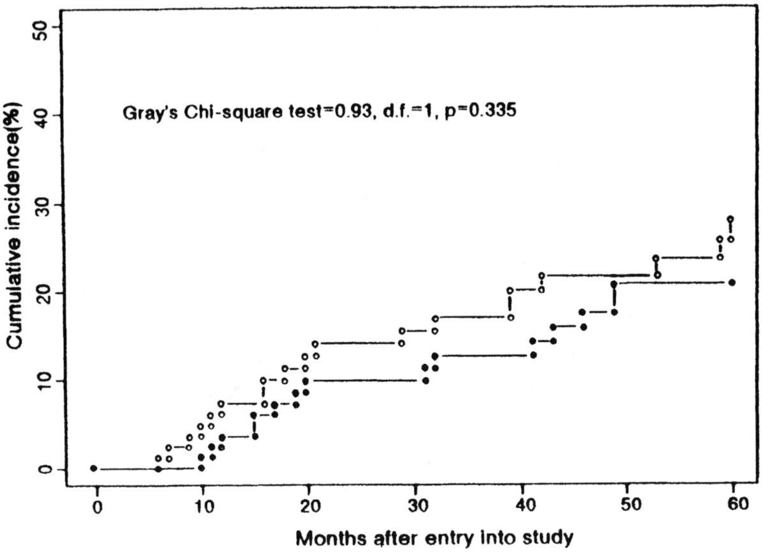

Fig. 2. Cumulative incidence of HCC in the 184 patients with AFP levels below 20 ng/ml at entry. ●: trial group (n = 93); ○: control group (n = 91).

(75%) than for the control group (61%) (p = 0.053). Figure 6 shows the cumulative survival curves of the patients without HBsAg. The survival curve for the trial group (76%) was significantly higher than that for the control group (60%) (p = 0.043).

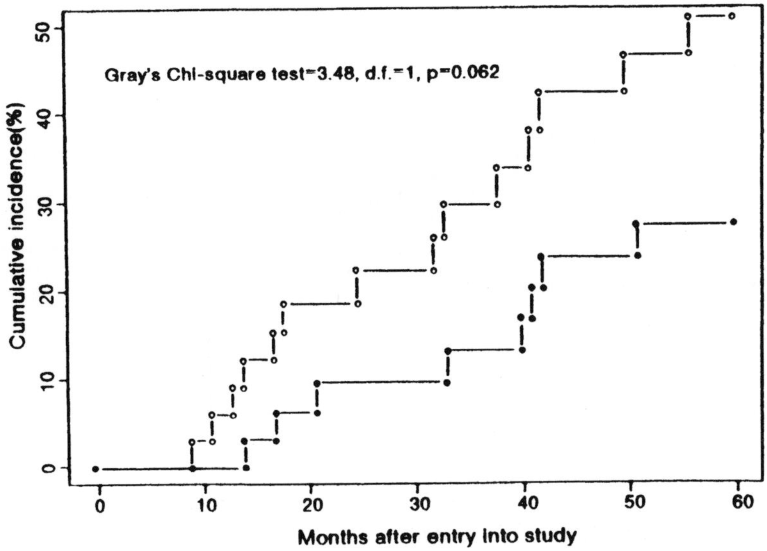

Fig. 3. Cumulative incidence of HCC in the 69 patients who had AFP levels between 20 and 200 ng/ml at entry. ●: trial group (n = 34); ○: control group (n = 35).

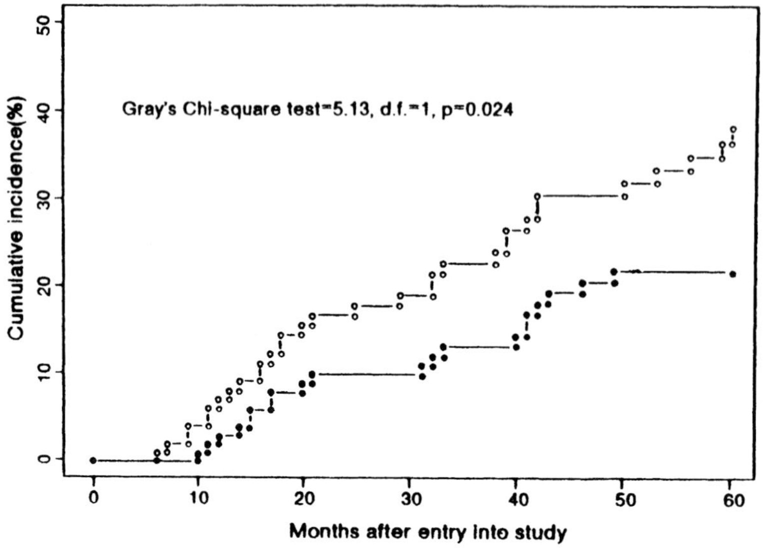

Fig. 4. Cumulative incidence of HCC in patients without HBs antigen. ●: trial group (n = 111); ○: control group (n = 106).

Discussion

This study is, to our knowledge, the first completed randomized controlled prospective trial of chemoprevention of HCC. The addition of TJ-9 had a positive

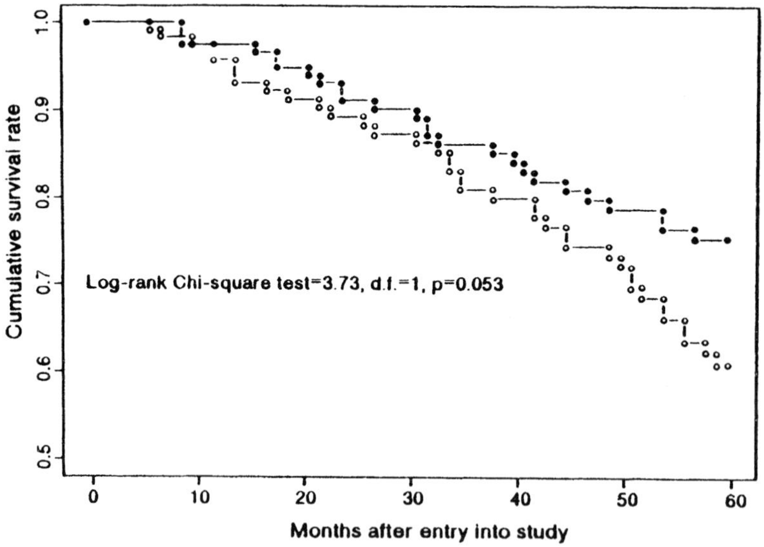

Fig. 5. Cumulative survival rate of the patients with cirrhosis in the two groups. ●: trial group (n = 127); ○: control group (n = 126).

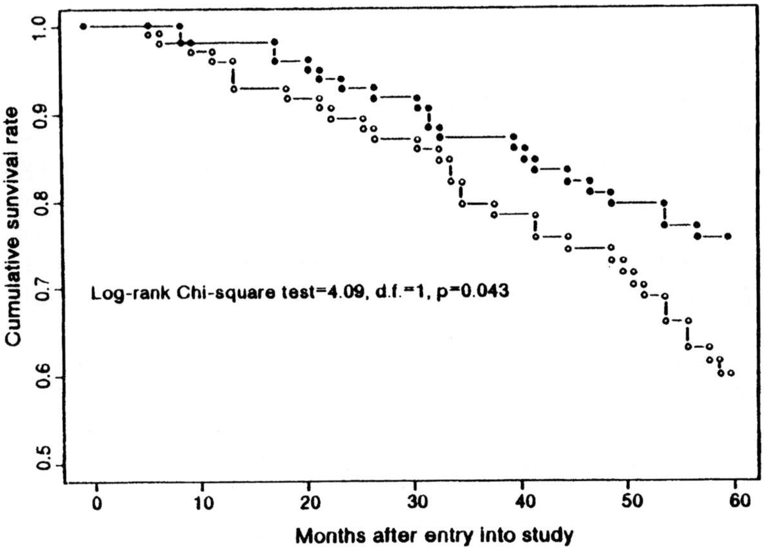

Fig. 6. Cumulative survival rate of the patients negative for HBs Ag. ●: trial group (n = 111); ○: control group (n = 106).

effect in both lowering the incidence of HCC and prolonging survival, but neither difference achieved statistical significance at $p < 0.05$.

The principles underlying Chinese herbal treatment were established in China over thousands of years on the basis of clinical experience and practice, but the effective ingredients usually have not been identified. TJ-9 is a Chinese herbal medicine used widely in Japan for the treatment of liver disease. In 7.5 g of TJ-9, there is 4.5 g of a dried TJ-9 extract, which is a dried concoction of seven herbs

Table 3. Ingredients of TJ-9.

Herbs	Weight (g)	Active ingredients
Bupleurum root	7.0	Saikosaponin-a Saikosaponin-b_1,b_2 Saikosaponin-c Saikosaponin-d
Pinellia tuber	5.0	L-ephedrine
Scutellaria root	3.0	Baicalin Baicalein
Jujube root	3.0	Cyclic AMP
Ginseng root	3.0	Ethyl-α-D-fructofuranoside
Glycyrrhiza root	2.0	Glycyrrhizin
Ginger rhizome	1.0	6-gingerol 6-shogaol Zingerone

Amount in 7.5 g of the drug.

(Table 3). The concentrations of the presumably active components in the Japanese preparation are regulated.

Many studies about the effects of TJ-9 were reported. TJ-9 prevented the morphologic and histochemical changes usually caused by D-galactosamine in rats [8,9], by danazol in 24 patients with endometriosis [10]. TJ-9 inhibited hepatocyte necrosis caused by CCl_4 [11] in rats, and hepatic fibrosis caused by porcine serum or dimethyl-nitrosamine in rats [12]. Oral administration of TJ-9 increased the natural killer cell activity in mice [13]. Intraperitoneal administration of TJ-9 activated macrophages in terms of phagocytic and lysosomal enzyme activities in mice [14].

In a study of the antitumor activity of several herbal preparations, Haranaka et al. [15] reported that seven of 12 mice were completely cured when TJ-9 were given orally before and after transplantation of Ehrlich tumors. Ito and Shimura [16] reported that oral administration of TJ-9 has an antimetastatic effect on Lewis lung carcinoma in mice. Tatsuta et al. [17] reported that treatment with TJ-9 inhibits the development of preneoplastic and neoplastic lesions of the liver after treatment of rats with N-nitrosomorpholine. They found that the administration of TJ-9 significantly increases the proportion of lymphocytes that are helper T cells. Okita et al. [18] investigated the inhibition of the proliferation of the human hepatoma cell line HuH-7, which produces AFP, using six purified components of TJ-9 separately. Baicalein, baicalin, and saikosaponin-a inhibit the growth of HuH-7 cells dose-dependently in all stages of the cell cycle. The production of AFP by cells treated with baicalein or baicalin or saikosaponin-a decreases dose-dependently, and tumor cell growth is inhibited simultaneously. They suggested that apoptosis had a role in cell death in that experiment. Yano et al. [19] reported that TJ-9 suppresses the proliferation of the human hepatoma cell line KIM-1 and the cholangiocarcinoma cell line KMC-1. TJ-9 showed much stronger antiproliferative effects than any one of its active ingredients; there could be synergistic or additive effects of various ingredients. In addition, there could be unknown substances present in TJ-9 that also inhibit tumor cell proliferation.

Analysis of cell morphology, DNA and the cell cycle showed two possible modes of action of TJ-9 in suppressing the proliferation of carcinoma cells. It may cause apoptosis soon after exposure of the cell to the agent, and it may cause cells to remain in the G_0/G_1 phase after a certain period of exposure. The effects of TJ-9 are difficult to explain as the effect of a single ingredient.

In our earlier prospective study [5], patients entering the study with AFP levels greater than 20 ng/ml had a significantly higher incidence of HCC evolution than those with normal AFP levels. Tsukuma et al. [20] and Ikeda et al. [21] reported similar results about the relationship between the serum level of AFP and the incidence of HCC. In this study, patients entering with AFP levels >20 ng/ml, the incidence of HCC in those given TJ-9 for up to 5 years was lower than in the control group. However, in the group of patients who had AFP levels <20 ng/ml at entry no difference was found between the two groups.

We speculated that TJ-9 might have inhibited the growth of cancer cells in the subclinical stage, when the number of cancer cells in the subclinical stage were much smaller than that in the clinical stage. The lower incidence of HCC in the trial group of patients with higher AFP levels supports this speculation.

It is unknown why the cumulative incidence of HCC was significantly lower in the trial group than in the control group in the patients without HBsAg. Most of the patients without HBsAg seem to have anti-C-100-3 antibodies, so this result suggests that TJ-9 is particularly effective for patients with hepatitis C virus.

The higher survival rate of the cirrhotic patients in the trial group could mean that TJ-9 had beneficial effects on the clinical course of patients with cirrhosis in addition to its inhibitory effect on HCC development.

References

1. Kew MC, Popper H. Relationship between hepatocellular carcinoma and cirrhosis. Semin Liver Dis 1984;4:136–146.
2. Oka H, Kurioka N, Kim K, Kanno T, Kuroki T, Mizoguchi Y et al. Prospective study of early detection of hepatocellular carcinoma in patients with cirrhosis. Hepatology 1990;12:680–687.
3. Ikegami T, Sugiura N, Ebara M, Saisho H, Ohto M. Development and predictive factors of hepatocellular carcinoma in patients with chronic liver disease over a long follow-up period. Jpn J Gastroenterol 1994;91:1290–1300. (in Japanese)
4. Oka H, Yamamoto S, Kuroki T, Harihara S, Marumo T, Kim SR et al. Prospective study of chemoprevention of hepatocellular carcinoma with Sho-saiko-to (TJ-9). Cancer 1995;76:743–749.
5. Oka H, Tamori A, Kuroki T, Kobayashi K, Yamamoto S. Prospective study of α-fetoprotein in cirrhotic patients monitored for development of hepatocellular carcinoma. Hepatology 1994; 19:61–66.
6. Gaynor JJ, Feuer EJ, Tan CC, Wu DH, Little CR, Straus DJ et al. On the use of cause-specific failure and conditional failure probabilities: examples from clinical oncology data. J Am Stat Assoc 1993;88:400–409.
7. Gray RJ. A class of κ-sample tests for comparing the cumulative incidence of a competing risk. Ann Statist 1988;16:1141–1154.
8. Yamamoto K, Araki N, Ogawa K. Ultrastructural and ultracytochemical examination of the effects of preadministration of Xiao-Chai-Hu-Tang on hepatic disorders induced by D-galactosamine HCl. Acta Histochem Cytochem 1985;18:403–418.
9. Araki N, Noda T, Ogawa K. Cytochemical studies on the effect of intraperitoneal and oral administration of a traditional Chinese medicine (Sho-saiko-to) on the D-galactosamine-induced hepatic injury of rats. Acta Histochem Cytochem 1988;21:439–453.
10. Yaginuma T, Okamura T, Takeuchi T, Nishii O, Fujimori R. Preventive effect of traditional herbal medicine, Sho-saiko-to, on danazol-induced hepatic damage. Int J Gynecol Obstet 1989;29: 337–341.
11. Amagaya S, Hayakawa M, Ogihara Y, Fujiwara K. Effects of Sho-saiko-to and Dai-saiko-to on carbon tetrachloride-induced hepatic injury in rats. J Med Pharm Soc Wakan-Yaku 1988;5: 129–136.
12. Amagaya S, Hayakawa M, Ogihara Y, Fujiwara K. Effects of Sho-saiko-to and Dai-saiko-to on experimental hepatic fibrosis in rats. J Med Pharm Soc Wakan-Yaku 1988;5:137–145.
13. Kaga H, Ochiak H, Kurokawa M, Sakuragawa N. Effects of Kampohozais (Sho-saiko-to, Ninjin-to, Hochu-ekki-to and Juzen-daiho-to) on immune responses in mice. Acta Med Biol 1991; 39:161–167.
14. Kumazawa Y, Takimoto H, Miura S, Nishimura C, Yamada A, Kawakita T et al. Activation of murine peritoneal macrophages by intraperitoneal administration of a traditional Chinese her-

bal medicine, xiao-chai-hu-tang (Japanese name: Sho-saiko-to). Int J Immunopharmacol 1988;10:395–403.

15. Haranaka K, Satomi N, Sakurai A, Haranaka R, Okada N, Kobayashi M. Antitumor activities and tumor necrosis factors producibility of traditional Chinese medicines and crude drugs. Cancer Immunol Immunother 1985;20:1–5.
16. Ito H, Shimura K. Effects of a blended Chinese medicine, Xiao-Chai-Hu-Tang, on Lewis lung carcinoma growth and inhibition of lung metastasis, with special reference to macrophage activation. Jpn J Pharmacol 1986;41:307–314.
17. Tatsuta M, Iishi H, Baba M, Nakaizumi A, Uehara H. Inhibition by Xiao-chai-hu-tang (TJ-9) of development of hepatic foci induced by N-nitrosomorholine in Sprague-Dawley rats. Jpn J Cancer Res 1991;82:987–992.
18. Okita K, Li Q, Murakamio T, Takahashi M. Anti-growth effects with components of Sho-saiko-to (TJ-9) on cultured human hepatoma cells. Eur J Cancer Prev 1993;2:169–176.
19. Yano H, Mizoguchi A, Fukuda K, Haramaki M, Ogasawara S, Momosaki S et al. The herbal medicine Sho-saiko-to inhibits proliferation of cancer cell lines by inducing apoptosis and arrest at the G_0/G_1 phase. Cancer Res 1994;54:448–454.
20. Tsukuma H, Hiyama T, Tanaka S, Nakao M, Yabuuchi T, Kitamura T et al. Risk factors for hepatocellular carcinoma among patients with chronic liver disease. N Engl J Med 1993;328: 1797–1801.
21. Ikeda K, Saitoh S, Koida I, Arase Y, Tsubota A, Chayama K et al. A multivariate analysis of risk factors for hepatocellular carcinogenesis: a prospective observation of 795 patients with viral and alcoholic cirrhosis. Hepatology 1993;18:47–53.

Progress in Hepatology, Volume 3.
Hepatocellular Carcinoma.
M. Yamanaka, G. Toda and T. Tanaka, editors.

Chemoprevention of hepatocarcinogenesis by retinoids – basic mechanisms and clinical experiences

Hisataka Moriwaki, Yoshimune Shiratori, Masataka Okuno, Ichiro Yasuda and Yasutoshi Muto
First Department of Internal Medicine, Gifu University School of Medicine, Gifu, Japan

Abstract. Effects of retinoids on liver carcinogenesis are controversial in experimental animals, depending on the affinity of retinoid ligands with nuclear retinoid receptors such as retinoic acid receptor (RAR) and retinoid X receptor (RXR). Acyclic retinoid is one of the RXR ligands, induces differentiation of human hepatoma-derived cell lines and inhibits chemically induced liver cancer in rats as well as spontaneous hepatoma in mice. A randomized controlled clinical trial demonstrated the preventive effect of the compound on the development of second primary tumors in patients with hepatocellular carcinoma. This effect is exerted by the deletion of premalignant or malignant clones by the retinoid. Basic mechanisms, clinical experiences and future application of retinoids for chemoprevention of hepatoma are reviewed.

Keywords: cancer chemoprevention, clonal deletion, differentiation induction, α-fetoprotein, hepatocellular carcinoma, retinoid.

Introduction

Retinoid is collectively termed as vitamin A (retinol) and its derivatives. Thousands of compounds are established including natural and synthetic retinoids (Fig. 1). Retinoid has a variety of functions such as growth promotion, maintenance of reproduction and dark adaptation. Retinoid also regulates cell differentiation and tissue morphogenesis. Since abnormality in the differentiation induces cellular atypia and that of the morphogenesis induces structural atypia, retinoid has important effects which inhibit carcinogenesis.

It is well known that hepatoma arises from chronic liver diseases associated with viral infection or alcohol. Abnormal metabolism of retinoids was revealed in hepatocarcinogenesis. Furthermore, not only experimental but also clinical studies suggest that repairs of these abnormalities may suppress hepatocarcinogenesis.

In this article, basic mechanisms, clinical experiences and future application of retinoids for chemoprevention of hepatoma are reviewed.

Address for correspondence: Hisataka Moriwaki MD PhD, First Department of Internal Medicine, Gifu University School of Medicine, 40 Tsukasa-machi, Gifu 500, Japan.

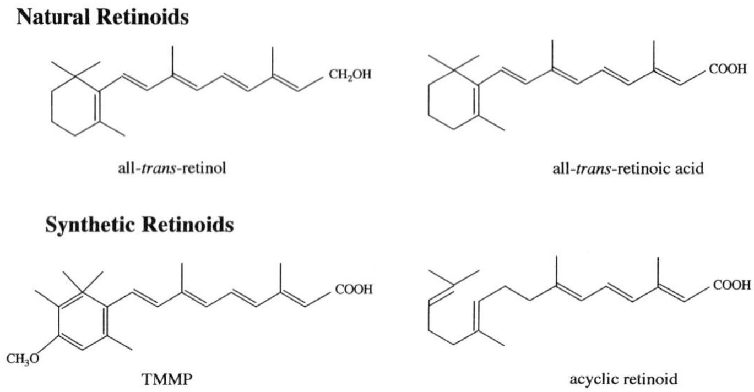

Fig. 1. Chemical structures of typical natural and synthetic retinoids.

Altered retinoid metabolism in hepatocarcinogenesis

In the analysis of retinoid concentration in the tissue of human and experimental hepatomas, it was shown that the concentration is reduced in premalignant and malignant lesions [1—4]. It is suggested that premalignant and malignant tissues loose (or catabolize) retinoids which suppress hepatocarcinogenesis [4].

Cellular retinoid-binding proteins also show remarkable changes in malignant tissues. Cellular retinol-binding protein levels are greatly reduced, whereas cellular retinoic acid-binding protein and cellular retinoid-binding protein, F-type, which is an onco-fetal protein, newly appeared [2].

Recent findings suggest that hepatocarcinogenesis involves alteration in nuclear retinoid receptors. The nuclear retinoid receptors are members of the steroid/thyroid hormone/vitamin D receptor family. There are two types of retinoid nuclear receptors: retinoic acid receptors (RAR) and retinoid X receptors (RXR). Each of the receptor types has at least three subtypes: α, β and γ. Since they act as ligand-activated *trans*-acting transcription factors and mediate the effects of retinoids on gene expression, abnormality in nuclear retinoid receptors may associate with abnormal gene expression in the carcinogenesis process.

There is a famous story of altered nuclear retinoid receptors in the carcinogenesis process, that is the produce of fusion protein of RAR with PML in acute promyelocytic leukemia [5]. The functional abnormality of altered RAR is repaired by giving all-trans retinoic acid (ATRA), a native ligand for RAR, which is the mechanism of the differentiation induction therapy in this leukemia [6].

Recently, we have found that there is also an alteration of RXR in hepatocarcinogenesis [7,8]. It is well-known that RXR is more important than RAR for the induction of cell differentiation or mutuality in hepatocyte [9]. Thereby, the mechanism of suppression of hepatocarcinogenesis by the retinoids which have high affinity with RXR may be explained by the same concept, that the functional abnormality of altered receptor is repaired by its native ligand.

Basic mechanisms of suppression of hepatocarcinogenesis by retinoids

Hepatoma arises from chronic viral or alcoholic liver diseases. The livers with these chronic diseases are likely to have multiple and independent clones of premalignant cells. These clones develop multicentric carcinogenesis. Such a characteristic pattern of carcinogenesis is explained by a concept of field cancerization which postulates that multiple cancers arise from a field that is exposed to continuous carcinogenic insults [10]. In order to prevent hepatocarcinogenesis in liver cirrhosis or recurrence as a second primary hepatoma after curative treatments, deletion and/or inhibition of such clones is essential [11]. Clonal deletion is realized by deletion of premalignant cells in the promotion, conversion or progression phase and clonal inhibition is realized by inhibition of development of transformed cells to the next phase.

The retinoid deletes premalignant or malignant clones by two possible mechanisms. One mechanism is that the cascade of transcription factors induce the differentiation of premalignant or malignant clones, through a signal that begins with the binding of the retinoid to the RXR [9]. It is followed by the recovery of programmed cell death, and premalignant clones must be finally deleted. The other mechanism is that, in a short period, the retinoid causes apoptosis which does not accompany the differentiation, also premalignant clones are completely deleted [12]. This mechanism does not require well-known receptors such as RAR and RXR [13] and is speculated as that apoptosis in hepatoma is caused by blocking the autocrine and paracrine loops of transforming growth factor α.

Clinical effect of retinoid on hepatocarcinogenesis

Effects of retinoids including natural and synthetic compounds on carcinogenesis have been investigated in a variety of animal models of hepatoma. However, these results have a lot of varieties including suppression, no change, and activation [14]. It may be explained that the effect of each compound associates with their binding specificities to nuclear receptors such as RAR and RXR.

In attempts to develop novel synthetic compounds for cancer chemoprevention, we found a 20-carbon polyprenoic acid [3,7,11,15-tetramethyl-2,4,6,10,14-hexadecapentaenoic acid] (Fig. 1) that binds to the cellular retinoic acid-binding protein and has relatively low toxicity [15]. This agent suppresses cell growth and the production of α-fetoprotein (AFP) and induces cell differentiation [9] and apoptosis [12,13] in human hepatoma-derived cell lines. Furthermore, it inhibits chemically induced hepatocarcinogenesis in rats [15] and spontaneous hepatoma in mice [4]. Its action is mediated in part through RAR and RXR [9]. This compound is called an open chain or acyclic retinoid.

All cirrhotic patients have a high risk since the annual incidence of primary hepatomas in these patients is 7 or 8%. Moreover, the patients who received the curative treatment of the initial hepatoma have a higher incidence of second primary hepatomas at 20 to 25% a year. We conducted a randomized controlled study to test whether polyprenoic acid prevents second primary hepatomas, which associate with multicentric carcinogenesis, after curative surgical resection or the percutaneous injection of ethanol into the initial hepatoma [16]. As compared with placebo, 12 months administration of polyprenoic acid prevented second primary hepatomas significantly (Fig. 2) [16].

In this clinical study, we also demonstrated that abnormal clone was suppressed and/or eradicated by the retinoid by measuring an isoform of serum AFP as a possible marker of the clone. AFP has a microheterogeneity due to structural variations in its sugar chain [20,21]. AFP-L3, an isoform of AFP, is reactive with lens culinaris agglutinin and is known to suggest the presence of latent hepatoma cells in the cirrhotic liver [22—24] and in the remnant liver after the curative removal of preceding hepatoma [25]. This result shows that the abnormal clone which produces AFP-L3 received clonal suppression as well as clonal deletion (Fig. 3) [17], suggesting that basic mechanism of suppression of hepatocarcinogenesis by retinoids as described earlier is realized in clinical cases.

Future directions

The most important target for suppression of hepatocarcinogenesis is to reduce the carrier rate of hepatitis virus.

In order to prevent hepatocarcinogenesis in patients with chronic liver disease, we can choose antivirus therapy by interferon-α [18] anti-inflammatory therapy by Sho-saiko-to [19], as well as chemoprevention by retinoid. We expect the theoretical strategy to prevent hepatocarcinogenesis by retinoid in the steps of carcinogenesis is applicable for other cancers.

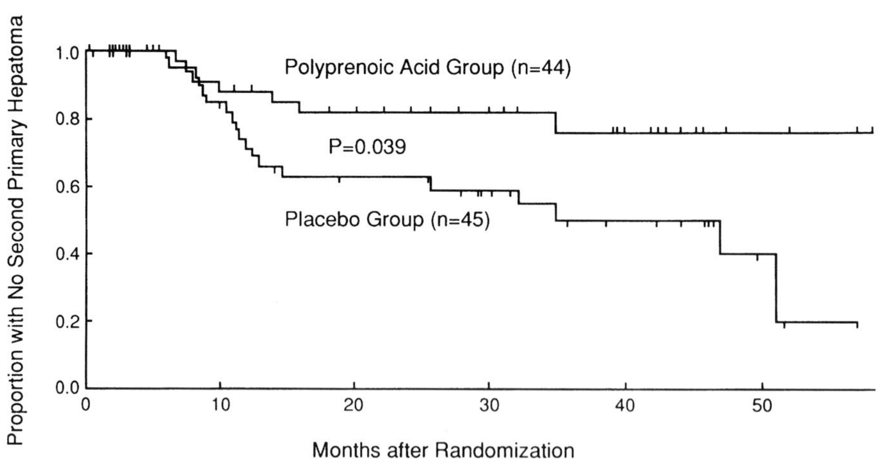

Fig. 2. Kaplan-Meier estimates of the proportion of patients without second primary hepatomas in the two study groups [16]. The treatment period lasted for 12 months, beginning at month 0; p = 0.04 for the comparison between groups by the log-rank test.

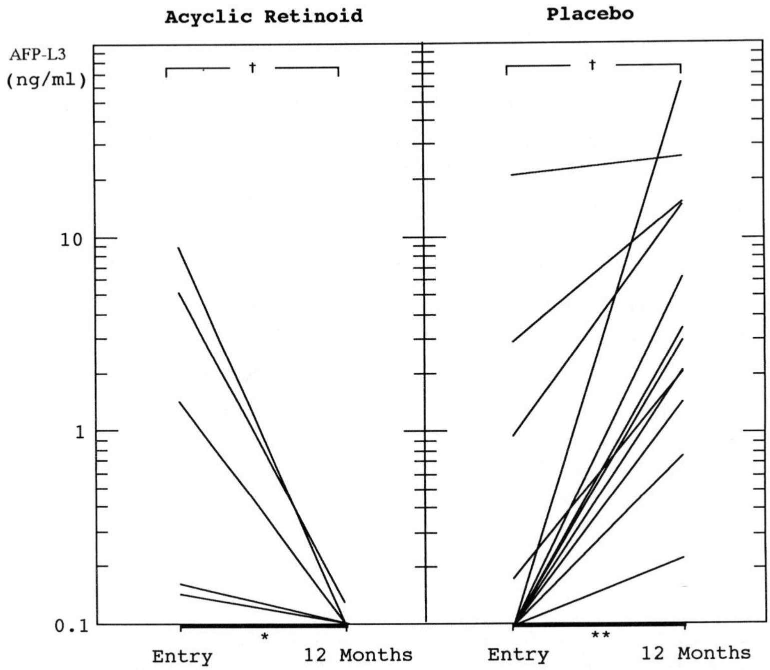

Fig. 3. Serum AFP-L3 levels at entry and after 12-month therapy in the acyclic retinoid group (left panel) and in the placebo group (right panel) [17]. †$p < 0.01$ by the paired t test; *serum AFP-L3 in 16 patients in the acyclic retinoid group; **9 patients in the placebo group remained below the detection range.

References

1. Muto Y, Omori M, Sugawara K. Demonstration of a novel cellular retinol-binding protein, F-type, in hepatocellular carcinoma. Jpn J Cancer Res (GANN) 1979;70:215–222.
2. Moriwaki H, Muto Y, Ninomiya M et al. Time course of changes in cellular retinoid-binding proteins in liver hyperplastic nodules and hepatocellular carcinoma experimentally induced in rats. Acta Hepatol Jpn 1982;55:523–529.
3. Muto Y, Kawai K, Moriwaki H. Antitumor activity of a novel synthetic polyprenoic acid (E5166) on "spontaneous" hepatic tumors of C3H/HeNCrj mice. In: Saurat JH (ed) Retinoids: New Trends in Research and Therapy. Basel: Karger, 1985;293–297.
4. Muto Y, Moriwaki H. Antitumor activities of vitamin A and its derivatives. J Natl Cancer Inst 1984;73:1389–1393.
5. de The H et al. The t(15;17) translocation of acute promyelocytic leukemia fuses the retinoic acid receptor alpha gene to a novel transcribed locus. Nature 1990;347:558–561.
6. Huang ME, Ye YC, Chen SR et al. Use of all-trans retinoic acid in the treatment of acute promyelocytic leukemia. Blood 1988;72:567–572.
7. Matsushima-Nishiwaki R, Shidoji Y, Nishiwaki S et al. Aberrant metabolism of retinoid X receptor proteins in human hepatocellular carcinoma. Mol Cell Endocrinol 1996;121:179–190.
8. Matsushima-Nishiwaki R, Shidoji Y, Nishiwaki S et al. Limited degradation of retinoid X receptor by calpain. Biochem Biophys Res Commun 1996;225:946–951.
9. Yamada Y, Shidoji Y, Fukutomi Y et al. Positive and negative regulations of albumin gene expression by retinoids in human hepatoma cell lines. Mol Carcinogenesis 1994;10:151–158.

10. Slaughter PD, Southwick HW, Smejkel W. "Field cancerization" in oral stratified epithelium: clinical implications of multicentric cancer. Cancer 1953;6:963–968.
11. Hong WK, Lippman SM, Hittelman WN et al. Retinoid chemoprevention of aerodigestive cancer: from basic research to the clinic. Clin Cancer Res 1995;1:677–686.
12. Nakamura N, Shidoji Y, Yamada Y, Hatakeyama H, Moriwaki H, Muto Y. Induction of apoptosis by acyclic retinoid in the human hepatoma-derived cell line, HuH-7. Biochem Biophys Res Comm 1995;207:382–388.
13. Nakamura N, Shidoji Y, Moriwaki H et al. Apoptosis in human hepatoma cell line by 4,5-didehydro geranylgeranoic acid (acyclic retinoid) via downregulation of transforming growth factor-α. Biochem Biophys Res Comm 1996;219:100–104.
14. Moon RC, Mehta RG, Rao KVN. Retinoids and cancer in experimental animals. In: Sporn MB, Roberts AB, Goodman DS (eds) The Retinoids: Biology, Chemistry, and Medicine, 2nd edn, New York: Raven Press, 1994;573–595.
15. Moriwaki H et al. Inhibitory effects of synthetic acidic retinoid and polyprenoic acid on the development of hepatoma in rats induced by 3′-methyl-N, N-dimethyl-4-aminoazobenzene. J Gastroenterol (Gastroenterol Jpn) 1988;23:546–552.
16. Muto Y, Moriwaki H et al. Prevention of second primary tumors by an acyclic retinoid, polyprenoic acid, in patients with hepatocellular carcinoma. N Engl J Med 1996;334:1561–1567.
17. Moriwaki H et al. Deletion of serum lectin-reactive alpha-fetoprotein by acyclic retinoid: a potent biomarker in the chemoprevention of second primary hepatoma. Clin Cancer Res (in press).
18. Nishiguchi S et al. Randomized trial of effects of interferon-alpha on incidence of hepatocellular carcinoma in chronic active hepatitis C with cirrhosis. Lancet 1995;346:1051–1055.
19. Oka H et al. Prospective study of chemoprevention of hepatocellular carcinoma with Sho-saiko-to (TJ-9). Cancer 1995;76:743–749.
20. Aoyagi Y, Suzuki Y, Isemura M, Nomoto M, Sekiya C, Igarashi K, Ichida F. The fucosylation index of alpha-fetoprotein and its usefulness in the early diagnosis of hepatocellular carcinoma. Cancer 1988;61:769–774.
21. Taketa K, Sekiya C, Namiki M, Akamatsu K, Ohta Y, Endo Y, Kosaka K. Lectin-reactive profiles of alpha-fetoprotein characterizing hepatocellular carcinoma and related conditions. Gastroenterology 1990;99:508–518.
22. Sato Y, Nakata K, Kato Y, Shima M, Ishii N, Koji T, Taketa K, Nagataki S. Early recognition of hepatocellular carcinoma based on altered profiles of alpha-fetoprotein. N Engl J Med 1993; 328:1802–1806.
23. Taketa K, Endo Y, Sekiya C, Tanikawa K, Koji T, Taga H, Satomura S, Matsuura S, Kawai T, Hirai H. A collaborative study for the evaluation of lectin-reactive a-fetoproteins in early detection of hepatocellular carcinoma. Cancer Res 1993;53:5419–5423.
24. Shiraki K, Takase K, Tameda Y, Hamada M, Kosaka Y, Nakano T. A clinical study of lectin-reactive alpha-fetoprotein as an early indicator of hepatocellular carcinoma in the follow-up of cirrhotic patients. Hepatology 1995;22:802–807.
25. Yamashita F, Tanaka M, Satomura S, Tanikawa K. Prognostic value of lens culinaris agglutinin-A-reactive α-fetoprotein in patients with hepatocellular carcinoma. Gastroenterology 1997;(in press).

Progress in Hepatology, Volume 3.
Hepatocellular Carcinoma.
M. Yamanaka, G. Toda and T. Tanaka, editors.

The prevention of hepatocellular carcinoma by the method of interferon therapy for chronic type C hepatitis

Yasuji Arase and Hiromitsu Kumada
Department of Gastroenterology, Toranomon Hospital, Tokyo, Japan

Abstract. Interferon (IFN) is effective in reducing serum alanine aminotransferase and in eliminating HCV in some patients with chronic hepatitis C. To explain the preventive effect of hepatocellular carcinoma (HCC) in patients treated with interferon (IFN) and to assess the risk factors for hepatocellular carcinogenesis, we studied 983 patients with chronic type C hepatitis for one to 7.6 years (median 2.8 years). Of these 983 patients, 324 (33%) showed a complete response with persistent HCV-RNA negativity for more than 6 months after completing IFN therapy. During the observation period, HCC developed in 32 patients. We divided the patients into four groups based on the effect of IFN: complete response, incomplete response, transient effective response and noneffective response. The cumulative appearance rate of HCC in complete response was less than that of noneffective response. Therefore, we conclude that the liver carcinogenesis could be inhibited by the IFN therapy in patients with chronic hepatitis C.

Keywords: chronic type C hepatitis, hepatitis C virus, hepatocellular carcinoma, interferon, laparoscopy.

Introduction

Interferon (IFN) treatment reduces the serum level of hepatitis C virus (HCV) [1–6]. However, there are a few reports about the appearance rates of hepatocellular carcinoma (HCC) after IFN therapy for chronic hepatitis C. Therefore we studied HCC appearance rates after IFN therapy in an effort to clarify which patient factors correlated with high HCC appearance rates, using Cox regression analysis.

Materials and Methods

Patients

From January 1988 to April 1995, 983 patients (786 males, 197 females) were enrolled in the trial; they were between 16 and 72 years old (median 46 years old). The enrollment criteria were: (1) the average ALT exceeded the upper limit of the normal range (6–50 IU) for more than 6 months before IFN; (2) liver biopsies within 6 months prior to IFN administration showed the histology of chronic liver disease, and the diagnosis was confirmed with both laparoscopy and liver biopsy; (3) detectable in serum using reverse transcription rested poly-

Address for correspondence: Dr Y Arase, Department of Gastroenterology, Toranomon Hospital, 2-2-2 Toranomon, Minato-ku, Tokyo 105, Tokyo, Japan.

merase chain reaction (RT-nested PCR) before IFN therapy; (4) no corticosteroid or other immunosuppressive agent administration 6 months before and/or during IFN treatment; (5) no hepatitis B surface antigens, hepatitis B virus DNA, antinuclear antibodies, antimitochondrial antibodies detectable in serum using radioimmununoassay and spot hybridization.

The follow-up started on the day IFN administration was completed. The IFN vials used contained 6∼10 MIU of IFN-α or IFN-β. Among the total of 983 patients, 592 received daily injections for 2 to 8 weeks, followed by IFN 2 or 3 times a week for another 16 weeks; 251 patients received injections 3 times a week for more than 24 weeks; and 140 patients received daily injections for 4 to 8 weeks. Complete responders (CR) were defined as those whose HCV-RNA was persistently negative for more than 6 months after completion of the IFN administration. Incomplete responders (ICR) were defined as those whose HCV-RNA was positive but ALT was normal after completion of the IFN therapy. Transient effective responders (TR) were those whose ALT was normal during IFN therapy and was relapsed after termination of the IFN. Lastly, noneffective responders (NR) were those except for CR, ICR and TR.

Follow-up

In patients treated with IFN, clinical evaluation and biochemical and hematological tests were performed at monthly intervals during follow-up. Thirty-one patients dropped out because of changes of address and employment between 0.3–7.2 years from the start of follow-up. These patients were dealt with as censored data in the following statistical analysis [7], because the eventual outcome in terms of HCC appearance could not be ascertained. Deaths unrelated to HCC were also classified as withdrawals and were regarded as censored cases. The median observation period for the entire patients group was 2.8 years (range 1–7.8 years). The diagnosis of HCC was based on typical hypervascular characteristics on angiography, in addition to specific computed tomographic and ultrasonographic features. Microscopic examination by fine-needle biopsy was performed in patients whose angiograms did not demonstrate atypical HCC image. Pathological confirmation using surgically resected specimens was carried out in 23 patients.

Examination of HCV-RNA and HCV serological groups

Serum samples were stored at $-80°C$ until analysis for HCV-RNA and HCV-serological grouping. The HCV-RNA was assayed using (RT-nested PCR). The HCV-serological group was classified by Kohara's method [8].

Liver histology and laparoscopic findings

Liver histology was classified, based on the extent of fibrosis, into four stages:

stage 1, periportal fibrosis expansion; stage 2, porto-portal septa; stage 3, porto-central linkage or bridging fibrosis; stage 4, cirrhosis. The laparoscopic findings were classified, based on irregularities of the liver surface, into three groups: smooth (and essentially smooth liver surface or with limited areas of depression); irregular (a liver surface showing increased number of small interconnected depression, possibly resembling ripples); nodular (a liver surface with nodular formations).

Statistical analysis

The appearance rates of HCC were analyzed by the log-rank test. A Cox proportional-hazards model was used to analyze factors contributing to the HCC appearance rates; the factors examined included age, sex, histological stage, laparoscopic findings, HCV-serological group, history of blood transfusion and effect of IFN. The analysis was conducted using a Biomedical Computer Program P(BMDP, University of California Press) [9,10].

Results

Of the 987 patients treated with IFN, 324 (33%) had CR, 98 (10%) had ICR, 255 (25.9%) had TR and 306 (31.1%) had NR. Figure 1 shows the cumulative HCC appearance rates according to the effectiveness of IFN therapy. The HCC appearance rates in NR were significantly higher than that in the other three responders (CR, ICR and TR) ($p<0.05$).

Risk factors for HCC

Cox regression analysis was performed with the seven variables mentioned in the Materials and Methods under Patients section.

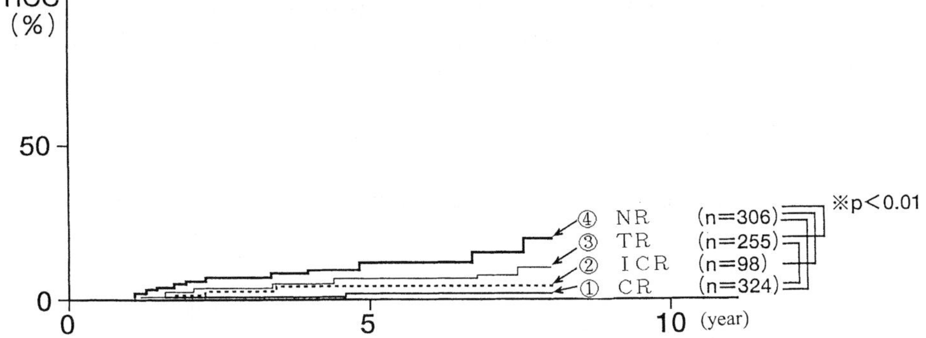

Fig. 1. Cumulative hepatocellular carcinoma (HCC) appearance rate based on the effectiveness of IFN therapy for chronic hapatitis C.

Univariate Cox regression analyses showed that the cumulative HCC appearance rate increased significantly when; (1) a nodular or 凹凸 liver surface was revealed by laparoscopy (p = 0.000) or the liver histology was stage 3 or 4 (p = 0.098), (2) IFN therapy was no CR (p = 0.022) (Table 1).

Because the variables were mutually correlated, multivariate Cox regression analysis was performed with the four statistically significant variables identified by the model. This analysis showed that the laparoscopic findings correlated most strongly with liver carcinogenesis during the short observation period. The relative risk in patients with 凹凸 or a nodular liver surface was 4.65, as compared with that of patients with a smooth or an irregular liver surface. The relative risk in patients who did not respond to IFN therapy was 2.98, compared to those who responded to IFN therapy.

Discussion

HCC is one of the most common cancers in the world. Recently, more than about 80% of patients with HCC were found to have RNA for the HCV [11]. The yearly incidence of HCC in patients with HCV-RNA positive cirrhosis ranges from 5 to 7% in Japan [11–13]. Kiyosawa et al. [14] reported that patients with long-term abnormal serum levels after transfusion had a high probability of histological aggravation as well as HCC. In Japan, long-term administration of Sho-sai-ko-to [15] or Stronger Neo-Minophagen C (SNMC) [16] against chronic liver disease type C was effective in preventing liver carcinogenesis. But these drugs have not got an antivirus effect directly. The reason why SNMC administration reduces hepatocarcinogenesis is believed to be related to the suppression of the necro-inflammatory reaction in the liver and the protection against histologic aggravation.

Recently, several authors have confirmed the therapeutic effects of IFN for chronic hepatitis C [1–6], but they were nearly all under 40–50%; the remaining cases had abnormal ALT levels. The aim of IFN therapy for chronic type C hepatitis is to reduce histological aggravation and liver carcinogenesis. We previously reported [17] that cases showing a complete response had the potential for histological improvement, and that IFN held promise of preventing the development of HCC in chronic hepatitis C.

Table 1. Factors associated with HCC appearance by Cox regression analysis.

Factors	Category	Odds ratio	95% CI	p value
Laparoscopic findings	1. smooth		1.28 ~ 4.67	0.000
	2. irregular. nodular	4.65		
Effects of IFN	1. response		1.25 ~ 10.38	0.022
	2. no response	2.98		
Histology	1. stage 1,2		1.46 ~ 3.32	0.098
	2. stage 3,4	2.25		

In this study, we investigated the appearance rates and predictive factors for HCC in chronic type C hepatitis over the short-term observation period after IFN therapy. It was apparent that laparoscopic findings are more useful than histology for predicting liver carcinogenesis. In fact, liver biopsy is a useful examination for assessing the type and severity of chronic liver disease. Thus, whether to use laparoscopy with liver biopsy remains a question. Harada [18] reported the significance of multiple liver biopsies in liver cirrhosis when the rates of histological diagnosis in two different parts of the liver coincided to the extent of 78.9%. Harada's results suggest that liver cirrhosis is not diagnosed accurately by liver biopsy alone. In the present study, approximately 20% of patients with a nodular liver surface were not diagnosed as having liver cirrhosis when only histological samples were used. In these patients, the HCC appearance rates were thought to be similar to those in patients diagnosed histologically as having liver cirrhosis.

Next, we are faced with the problem of the effectiveness of IFN therapy in terms of liver carcinogenesis. In this study, the relative risk of HCC in patients who did not respond to IFN therapy was almost 3 times that of patients who responded. Moreover, the appearance rate of HCC per year in IFN-treated patients is lower than that in IFN-untreated patients. Therefore IFN therapy appears to decrease the incidence of liver carcinogenesis. It is thought that the clearance of HCV and the control of hepatic inflammation achieved by IFN therapy contribute to the diminution of liver carcinogenesis.

References

1. Hoofnale JH, Mullen KD, Jones DB et al. Treatment of chronic non-A, non-B hepatitis with recombinant human alpha interferon. N Engl J Med 1986;315:1575–1578.
2. Kiyosawa K, Sodeyma S, Oike Y et al. Treatment of chronic non-A, non-B, hepatitis with human interferon-beta. In : Zuckerman A (ed) Viral Hepatitis and Liver Disease. New York: Alan R. Liss, 1988;898–901.
3. Chayama K, Saitoh S, Arase Y et al. Effect of interferon administration on serum hepatitis C virus RNA in patients with chronic hepatitis C. Hepatology 1991;13:1040–1043.
4. Arase Y, Chayama K, Tsubota A et al. Alanine aminotransferase and HCV-RNA responses following interferon therapy of HCV-RNA in positive chronic hepatitis. Gastroenterologic a Japonica 1992;27:646–651.
5. Tsubota A, Chayama K, Ikeda K et al. Factors predictive of response to interferon-alpha therapy in hepatitis C virus infection. Hepatology 1994;19:1088–1094.
6. Hino K, Sainokami S, Shimoda K et al. Genotype and titers of hepatitis C for predicting response to interferon in patients with chronic hepatitis C. J Med Virology 1994;42:299–305.
7. Harrington DP, Fleming TR. A class of rank test procedures for censored survival data. Biomedica 1982;62:553–566.
8. Tsukiyam-Kohara K, Yamaguchi K, Maki N et al. Antigenicities of group 1 and 11 hepatitis C virus polypeptides-molecular basis of diagnosis. Virology 1993;192:430–437.
9. Cox DR. Regression models and life tables. JR Stat Soc 1972;34:248–275.
10. Dixon WJ, Brown MB, Engleman L et al. BMDP Statistical Software. Berkeley: University of California, 1985.
11. Ikeda K, Saotoh S, Koida I et al. A multivariate analysis of risk factors for hepatocellular carci-

nogeneses: a prospective observation of 795 patients with viral and alcoholic cirrhosis. Hepatology 1993;18:47–53.

12. Oka H, Kurioka N, Kim K et al. Prospective study of early detection of hepatocellular carcinoma with cirrhosis. Hepatology 1990;12:680–687.
13. Ikegami T, Sugiura N, Ebara M et al. Development and predictive factors of hepatocellular carcinoma in patients with chronic liver disease over a long follow-up period (in Japanese). Jpn J Gastroenterol 1994;91:1290–1300.
14. Kiyosawa K, Sodeyama T, Tanaka E et al. Interrelationship of blood transfusion, non-A, non-B hepatitis and hepatocellular carcinoma: analysis by detection of antibody to hepatitis C virus. Hepatology 1990;12:671–675.
15. Oka H, Yamamoto S, Kuroki T et al. Prospective study of chemoprevention of hepatocellular carcinoma with sho-saiko-to. Cancer 1995;76:743–749.
16. Arase Y, Ikeda K, Murashima N et al. The long-term efficacy of glycyrrhizin in chronic hepatitis C patients. Cancer 1997;79:1494–1500.
17. Arase Y, Chayama K, Murashima N et al. A long-term prognosis after interferon therapy for chronic hepatitis C. Acta Hepatol Jpn 1996;37:145–151.
18. Harada T. Significance of multiple liver biopsies in chronic hepatitis and liver cirrhosis. Kanseikensindanhou Ishiyakusyupan 1979;59.
19. Arase Y, Murashima M, Chayama Y et al. The superiority of laparoscopic examination in predicting hepatocellular carcinoma after IFN therapy for chronic type C hepatitis. Digestive Endoscopy 1997;9(1):29–33.

Progress in Hepatology, Volume 3.
Hepatocellular Carcinoma.
M. Yamanaka, G. Toda and T. Tanaka, editors.

Experience in surgical resection for small hepatocellular carcinoma

Junji Yamamoto[1], Tomoo Kosuge[1], Kazuaki Shimada[1], Keiji Sano[1], Susumu Yamasaki[1], Tadatoshi Takayama[2] and Masatoshi Makuuchi[2]
[1]*Department of Surgery, National Cancer Center Hospital, Tokyo; and* [2]*Second Department of Surgery, Tokyo University School of Medicine, 7-3-1 Hongo, Bunkyo-ku, Tokyo 113, Japan*

Abstract. *Objective.* To analyze the effectiveness of surgical therapy as a treatment for small hepatocellular carcinoma (HCC), we reviewed patients who had three or fewer HCCs of 3 cm or smaller in diameter.

Background. Small HCC has been reported to be potentially curable by percutaneous ethanol injection therapy.

Methods. We reviewed the records of 147 patients who underwent primary hepatic resection for three or fewer HCCs of 3 cm or smaller in diameter.

Results. Operative blood loss was less than 1,000 ml in 91 (61.9%) patients and less than 2,000 ml in 131 (89.1%). Only 19 (12.9%) patients received a red blood cell transfusion perioperatively. Overall 1-, 3- and 5-year survival rates were 95.9, 88.7 and 69.2%, respectively. Incomplete resection, multiple tumors and combined liver cirrhosis predicted a poor prognosis after resection. As for recurrence after surgery, the 1-, 3- and 5-year cumulative recurrence rates were 20.1, 58.8 and 81.3%, respectively.

Conclusion. While survival after surgery has improved, postresection recurrence is frequent. Surgical treatment resulted in better long-term survival. Surgery is a safe and effective treatment which should be adopted as a first treatment of choice for patients with small HCCs.

Keywords: hepatocellular carcinoma, primary hepatic resection, prognostic factors, recurrence, small hepatocellular carcinoma, surgery, surgical therapy, survival.

Introduction

Increasing number of patients are being diagnosed with small hepatocellular carcinoma (HCC) among those with chronic liver diseases, due to the development of imaging diagnosis and early detection plans for this tumor [1—3]. There have been several surgical reports on small HCC smaller than 5 cm in diameter [4—6]. In this study, we reviewed patients who had three or fewer HCCs of 3 cm or smaller in diameter, since several reports have indicated that these are the criteria for the potentially curative treatment of HCC by percutaneous ethanol injection (PEI) [7,8].

Address for correspondence: Junji Yamamoto MD, Department of Surgery, National Cancer Center Hospital, 5-1-1 Tsukiji, Chuo-ku, Tokyo 104, Japan. Telephone: +81-3-3542-2511 (extension 7-225).

Patients and Methods

Between 1990 and 1994, 149 patients underwent primary hepatic resection for treatment of three or fewer HCCs of 3 cm or smaller in diameter at the National Cancer Center Hospital, Tokyo, Japan. Two patients were lost during follow-up. The case records of the remaining 147 patients were reviewed. Three patients (2.0%) died either within 1 month after surgery, or during the initial hospital stay. After surgery, the patients were followed at least every 3 months by measurement of serum alpha fetoprotein (AFP), ultrasound and computed tomography, and if necessary, hepatic angiography. The follow-up period, excluding the patients lost to postoperative mortality, ranged from 9.0 to 82.1 months, with a median of 47.7 months and a mean of 48.1 months. Patients without recurrence were followed for at least 22.1 months after surgery.

The case records of all of the patients were reviewed. The following factors were analyzed with reference to their prognostic significance in survival and recurrence: age, gender, status of hepatitis virus infection, associated liver cirrhosis, hepatic reserve according to Child's classification, also the number and size of the tumor(s). Cumulative rates of survival and recurrence were calculated by the Kaplan-Meier method; differences between the curves were assessed using the log-rank test.

Results

Clinicopathologic data

During the same 5-year period, 386 patients underwent primary hepatic resection for treatment of HCC at our hospital. The 149 patients with three or fewer tumors of 3 cm or smaller in diameter comprised 38.6% of these cases. Among the remaining patients, 158 (40.9%) had three or fewer tumors larger than 3 cm, nine (2.3%) had more than three tumors 3 cm or smaller in diameter, and 70 (18.1%) had more than three tumors larger than 3 cm in diameter. Men outnumbered women by 146 to 41. Overall, 28 (19%) patients carried hepatitis B virus, while 99 (69.3%) had hepatitis C virus. Eighty-five (57.8%) patients had solitary tumor, 48 (32.7%) had two tumors, and 14 (9.5%) had three tumors in the liver. Fifty-one (34.7%) patients had tumors smaller than or equal to 2 cm in diameter, and 96 (65.3%) had tumors larger than 2 cm. As for the histologic differentiation of the tumors, 33 (22.4%) patients had well-differentiated HCC, 59 (40.1%) had moderately differentiated HCC, and 17 (11.6%) had poorly differentiated HCC. Thirty-eight (25.9%) patients had totally necrotic tumors due to preoperative transarterial embolization (TAE). According to the Child-Pugh classification, 99 (67.3%) patients were in Class A and 48 (32.7%) were in Class B or C. Histologic examination of noncancerous liver parenchyma showed that only three (2%) patients had normal liver, 52 (35.4%) had chronic hepatitis, and 92 (62.6%) had liver cirrhosis.

The operative procedure included 104 (70.7%) limited resections, 25 (17.0%) subsegmentectomies, 16 (10.9%) segmentectomies, and two (1.4%) isolated caudate lobe resections. The operative blood loss was smaller than 1,000 ml in 91 (61.9%) patients, 1,000–2,000 ml in 40 (27.2%), 2,000–3,000 ml in 10 (6.8%), and more than 3,000 ml in six (4.1%), with an average of 1,080 ml. Nineteen (12.9%) patients received a red blood cell transfusion. The surgical margin was secured larger than 5 mm in 49 (33.3%) patients and 5 mm or smaller in 69 (46.9%). Sixteen (10.9%) patients underwent incomplete resections due to an involved surgical margin and 13 (8.8%) underwent debulking resection due to limited liver function.

Survival analysis

The overall 1-, 3- and 5-year survival rates including hospital mortality were 95.9, 88.7 and 69.2%, respectively (Fig. 1). As for the curative value of surgery, patients who underwent complete resection of the tumors showed significantly better survival than those who received noncurative surgery (Fig. 2). Age, gender, and state of hepatitis virus infection did not affect the postresection outcome. Although the tumor size did not affect the prognosis after surgery, the number of tumors had unfavorable effects on patient survival (Fig. 3). The survival rates were 98.0, 91.4 and 72.2% for Child's Class A, and 89.6, 80.8 and 62.6% for Classes B and C. When classified by noncancerous liver parenchyma, patients with chronic hepatitis showed significantly better survival rates than those with cirrhosis (Fig. 4).

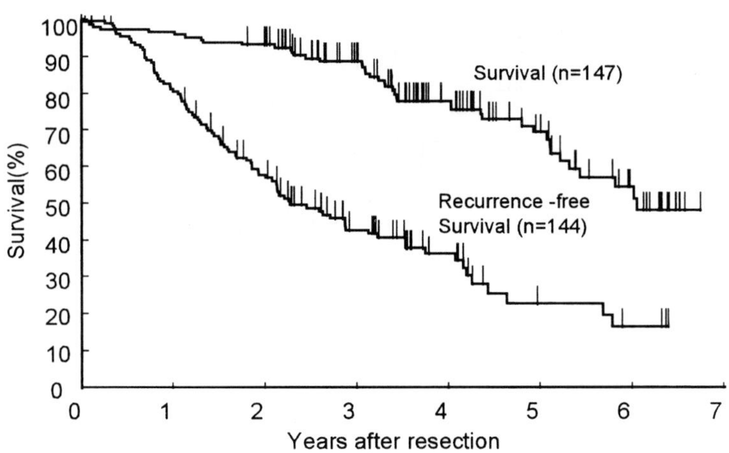

Fig. 1. Survival and recurrence-free survival after surgery. Cumulative survival and recurrence-free survival rates at 1, 3 and 5 years were 95.9, 88.7, 69.2, and 79.9, 41.2, 18.7%, respectively.

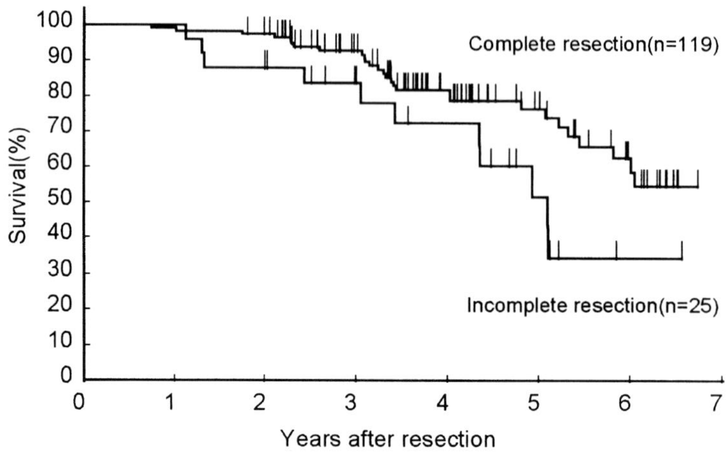

Fig. 2. Survival after complete and incomplete resection. Survival rates were 98.3, 92.8 and 76.5% at 1, 3 and 5 years, respectively, after complete resection, and 79.9, 41.2 and 18.7%, respectively, after incomplete resection. The difference was significant (p = 0.03).

Recurrence analysis

The 1-, 3- and 5-year cumulative recurrence-free survival rates were 89.9, 41.2 and 18.7%, respectively (Fig. 1). Incomplete resection and multiple tumors were significant unfavorable prognostic factors for postresection recurrence (Figs. 5 and 6).

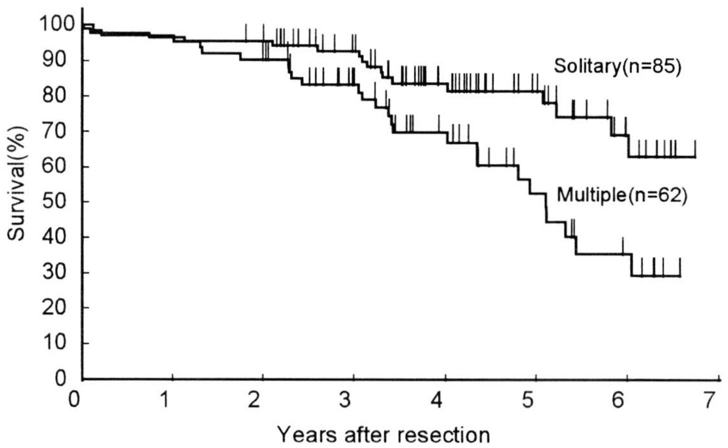

Fig. 3. Survival curve of the whole patients by the number of tumors. The patients with a solitary tumor showed significantly better outcome than those with multiple lesions (p = 0.002). Survival rates at 1, 3 and 5 years after surgery were 96.4, 92.7 and 81.6%, respectively, when the patients had a solitary tumor, and 96.8, 83.3 and 50.8%, respectively, when they had multiple lesions.

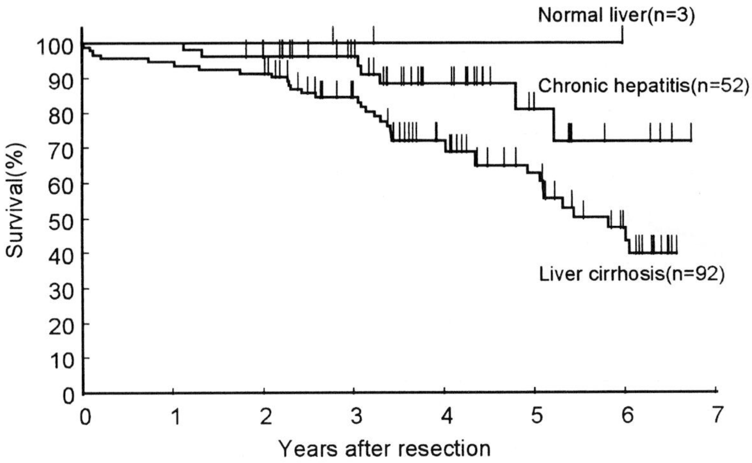

Fig. 4. Survival curve by associated liver diseases. The patients with chronic hepatitis demonstrated significantly better prognosis than those with liver cirrhosis ($p = 0.03$). The 1-, 3- and 5-year survival rate was 100, 96.2 and 80.9%, respectively, in patients with chronic hepatitis, and 94.6, 84.3 and 62.7%, respectively, in those with liver cirrhosis.

Discussion

The development of increasingly sensitive imaging techniques along with improved follow-up, treatment and screening of high-risk patients with chronic liver diseases has led to a change in the profile of patients with HCC. Before 1970, almost all HCC patients were symptomatic and had advanced diseases,

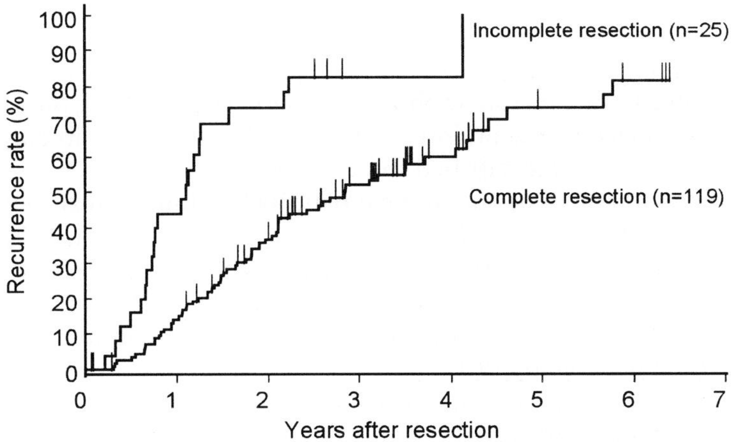

Fig. 5. Recurrence curve by completeness of resection. Incomplete resection was followed earlier and more frequent recurrences than complete resection ($p = 0.00003$). The cumulative recurrence rates were 14.0, 52.1 and 73.9%, respectively, in the patients who underwent complete resection, and 44.0, 82.5 and 100%, respectively, in those with incomplete resection.

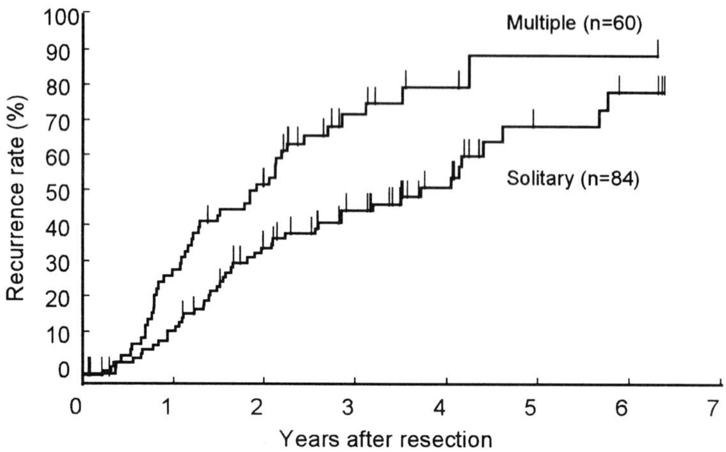

Fig. 6. Recurrence curve by the number of the tumors. The patients with multiple tumors developed significantly more frequent recurrence than those with a solitary lesion ($p = 0.0009$). Cumulative recurrence rates at 1, 3 and 5 years after surgery were 12.3, 46.5 and 70.6%, respectively, when the patients had a solitary tumor, and 29.3, 53.8 and 91.0%, respectively, when they had multiple lesions.

while there were many reports on subclinical or small HCCs in the 1980s [4—6]. Increasing numbers of reports on small HCCs in the early stage and a nodular hepatic lesions transformed to HCC have been published in the 1990s [10—13]. Investigations of the epidemiology, natural history and treatment strategies for HCC patients have been undertaken. Until the 1980s, the treatment of choice was surgical resection for single or a limited number of lesions and TAE with various anticancer agents for multiple lesions [14]. There have been several reports that surgery can offer better results than TAE in patients with small HCC [15,16]. Percutaneous ethanol injection (PEI) was developed in the late 1980s as another therapeutic option [7,8,17—22]. In some reports, the 3-year survival rates after PEI were comparable to or superior to those after surgery [18,19,23]. Since the criteria for PEI are ordinarily three or fewer tumors smaller than 3 cm in diameter [7,8], we analyzed patients who satisfied these criteria.

In this series, less than 40% of all of our surgical patients had tumors that met the criteria of PEI treatment. As for the background to liver parenchyma, 98% of the patients had viral hepatitis or cirrhosis after viral infection. The distribution of the Child-Pugh classification was also comparable to that of PEI-treated patients. As for the number of tumors, more patients in our series had multiple lesions (42.1%) than those undergoing PEI.

The patient outcome in our series was similar to that of previously reported in patients with surgically treated small HCC [5,6] but was superior to that of patients treated by PEI [18—23]. Even when we considered only patients with either liver cirrhosis or multiple tumors, the 3-year survival rates of our patients were far better than those treated by PEI. A comparison of the survival rates of patients who underwent curative and noncurative resection showed an advantage for complete resection. However, the 5-year survival rate of 51.8%, which is comparable to the 3-year survival rate of PEI-treated patients, suggests that initial resection therapy with subsequent adjunctive treatments would be reasonable for selected patients. Some researchers concluded that PEI gives results similar to those of surgery for the treatment of small HCCs, with a 3-year survival rate of 62 to 64%. However, they compared their results with the outcome of older surgical series [24–26], in which the diagnostic procedures were less accurate and perioperative mortality was higher than in more recent studies [27–29]. Decreased operative mortality is a major prerequisite for surgical treatment of HCC. In our study, operative mortality was 2.0%, which is comparable to that reported in a recent series [27–29]. About 90% of our patients underwent surgery with blood loss of less than 2,000 ml, and 87% of our patients did not receive a red blood cell transfusion.

In our series, surgery gave better long-term survival than PEI. The overall 5-year survival rate of around 70% was comparable to the 3-year survival rate reported for PEI-treated patients [8–23]. There have been few reports on PEI which discussed the long-term results (5 years or more) after treatment [19,21].

Despite the improved survival after surgery, however, postresection recurrence was frequent, due to early spread via the portal venous system as well as possible multicentric carcinogenesis of HCC. A marked difference between the cumulative rate of survival and recurrence indicated the effectiveness of postrecurrence treatment, such as repeated resection, TAE, and PEI. Our results suggest that surgery is an effective treatment which should be adopted as the first treatment of choice for patients with small HCCs.

Acknowledgements

This study was supported by a Grant-in-Aid for Cancer Research from the Ministry of Health and Welfare of Japan.

References

1. Okuda K, Kotoda K, Obata H et al. Clinical observation during a relatively early stage of hepatocellular carcinoma with special reference to alpha-fetoprotein levels. Gastroenterology 1975; 69:116–134.
2. Sheu JC, Sung JL, Chen DS et al. Ultrasonography of small hepatic tumors using high-resolution linear-array real-time instruments. Radiology 1984;150:797–802.
3. Okazaki N, Yoshida T, Yoshino M. Screening of patients with chronic liver disease for hepatocellular carcinoma by ultrasonography. Clin Oncol 1984;10:241–246.
4. Chen DS, Sheu JC, Sung JL et al. Small hepatocellular carcinoma-A clinicopathological study in thirteen patients. Gastroenterology 1982;83:1109–1119.
5. Tang ZY, Yu YQ, Zhou XD, Zhou NQ. Surgical treatment of subclinical hepatocellular carcinoma (HCC) and its ultimate outcome. A comparative study of 74 cases of subclinical HCC and 229 cases of clinical HCC undergone surgery. J Exp Clin Cancer Res 1983;3:261–268.
6. Hsu HC, Sheu JC, Lin YH et al. Prognostic histologic features of resected small hepatocellular carcinoma(HCC) in Taiwan. A comparison with resected large HCC. Cancer 1985;56:672–680.

7. Ebara M, Kita K, Yoshikawa M et al. Percutaneous ethanol injection for patients with small hepatocellular carcinoma. In: Tobe T et al. (eds) Primary Liver Cancer in Japan. Tokyo: Springer-Verlag, 1992;291–300.
8. Vilana R, Bruix J, Bru C, Ayuso C, Sole M, Rodes J. Tumor size determines the efficacy of percutaneous ethanol injection for the treatment of small hepatocellular carcinoma. Hepatology 1992;16:353–357.
9. Kanai T, Hirohashi S, Upton MP et al. Pathology of small hepatocellular carcinoma. A proposal for a new gross classification. Cancer 1987;60:810–819.
10. Takayama T, Makuuchi M, Hirohashi S et al. Malignant transformation of adenomatous hyperplasia to hepatocellular carcinoma. Lancet 1990;336:1150–1153.
11. Tuda H, Hisohashi S, Shimosato Y, Terada M, Hasegawa H. Clonal origin of atypical adenomatous hyperplasia of the liver and clonal identity with hepatocellular carcinoma. Gastroenterology 1988;95:1664–1666.
12. Rim K-S, Sakamoto M, Watanabe H et al. Pathology and DNA cytophotometry of small hepatocellular carcinoma with a nodule-in-nodule appearance. Evidence for stepwise progression of hepatocellular carcinoma. Jpn J Clin Oncol 1992;23:26–33.
13. Nakanuma Y, Terada T, Ueda K, Terasaki S, Nonomura A, Matsui O. Adenomatous hyperplasia of the liver as a precancerous lesion. Liver 1993;13:1–9.
14. Okuda K. Primary liver cancer: quadrennial review lecture. Dig Dis Sci 1986;31:133s–146s.
15. Kanematsu T, Matsumata T, Shirabe K et al. A comparative study of hepatic resection and transcatheter arterial embolization for the treatment of primary hepatocellular carcinoma. Cancer 1993;71:2181–2186.
16. Yamamoto K, Masuzawa M, Kato M, Okuyama T, Tamura K. Analysis of prognostic factors in patients with hepatocellular carcinoma treated by transcatheter arterial embolization. Cancer Chemother Pharmacol 1992;31(Suppl):S77–S81.
17. Sugiura N, Takara K, Ohto M et al. Treatment of small hepatocellular carcinoma by percutaneous injection of ethanol into tumor with real-time ultrasound monitoring. Acta Hepatol Jpn 1983;24:920.
18. Livraghi T, Bolondi L, Lazzaroni S et al. Percutaneous ethanol injection in the treatment of hepatocellular carcinoma in cirrhosis: a study on 207 patients. Cancer 1992;69:925–929.
19. Shiina S, Tagawa K, Niwa Y et al. Percutaneous ethanol injection therapy for hepatocellular carcinoma: results in 146 patients. AJR 1993;160:1023–1028.
20. Lencioni R, Bartolozzi C, Caramella D et al. Treatment of small hepatocellular carcinoma with percutaneous ethanol injection. Analysis of prognostic factors in 105 Western patients. Cancer 1995;76:1737–1746.
21. Livraghi T, Giorgio A, Marin G et al. Hepatocellular carcinoma and cirrhosis in 746 patients: long-term results of percutaneous ethanol injection. Radiology 1995;197:101–108.
22. Castells A, Bruix J, Bru C et al. Treatment of small hepatocellular carcinoma in cirrhotic patients: a cohort study comparing surgical resection and percutaneous ethanol injection. Hepatology 1993;18:1121–1126.
23. Livraghi T, Bolondi L, Buscarini L et al. No treatment, resection and ethanol injection in hepatocellular carcinoma: a retrospective analysis of survival in 391 patients with cirrhosis. J Hepatol 1995;22:522–526.
24. Nagasue N, Yukaya N, Okawa Y, Chang Y, Niimi K. Clinical experience with 118 hepatic resection for hepatocellular carcinoma. Surgery 1986;99:694–701.
25. Nagao T, Inoue S, Goto S et al. Hepatic resection for hepatocellular carcinoma. Clinical features and long-term prognosis. Ann Surg 1987;205:33–40.
26. Takayasu K, Muramatsu Y, Moriyama N. Clinical and radiologic assessments of the results of hepatectomy for small hepatocellular carcinoma and therapeutic arterial embolization for postoperative recurrence. Cancer 1989;64:1848–1852.
27. Makuuchi M, Kosuge T, Takayama T et al. Surgery for small liver cancers. Semin Surg Oncol 1993;9:298–304.

28. Ikeda K, Saitoh S, Tsubota A et al. Risk factors for tumor recurrence and prognosis after curative resection of hepatocellular carcinoma. Cancer 1993;71:19–25.
29. Di Carlo V, Ferrari G, Castoldi R et al. Surgical treatment and prognostic variables of hepatocellular carcinoma in 122 cirrhotics. Hepatogastroenterology 1995;42:222–229.

Progress in Hepatology, Volume 3.
Hepatocellular Carcinoma.
M. Yamanaka, G. Toda and T. Tanaka, editors.

Prognosis of patients with small hepatoma after percutaneous injection of ethanol

Masatoshi Tanaka, Masahiro Shimada, Noriyuki Ono, Yukio Tateishi, Yoshihiro Shimauchi, Ryoko Kuromatsu, Hitoshi Fukuda, Taku Kusaba, Shigeru Yutani and Kyuichi Tanikawa
Second Department of Internal Medicine, Kurume University School of Medicine, Kurume 830, Japan

Abstract. *Background/Aims.* Because of its efficacy and low incidence of complications, ethanol injection is widely used in Japan for treating patients with small hepatocellular carcinoma. We evaluated the long-term prognosis of 349 such patients and determined the prognostic variables having statistical significance.

Methods. We studied 349 patients with small (< 3 cm) hepatocellular carcinoma who received percutaneous injection of ethanol initially between April 1, 1984 and December 28, 1993. The prognosis was assessed by Kaplan-Meier method, and Cox's multivariate analysis was used to identify significant prognostic variables.

Results. Cumulative survival rates at 3, 5 and 7 years were 73.5, 47.0 and 27.0%, respectively. Significant prognostic variables were age, Child's classification, tumor histology, tumor size, and regular follow-up. Those with the greatest effect on survival were regular follow-up ($p<0.0001$) and tumor histology ($p<0.0001$).

Conclusions. Regular follow-up as well as the differentiation of hepatocellular carcinoma contributed to an improved survival rate of patients with small hepatocellular carcinoma following the percutaneous administration of ethanol.

Keywords: Child's classification, hepatocellular carcinoma, percutaneous ethanol injection therapy, prognostic variables, regular follow-up, small hepatocellular carcinoma, tumor histology, tumor size, ultrasonography.

Introduction

Hepatocellular carcinoma (HCC) is common among the Japanese. Periodic use of real-time ultrasonography (US) in patients with chronic hepatitis and liver cirrhosis often leads to the identification of small space hepatic lesions [1] which are diagnosed as HCC by US-guided tumor biopsy [2]. Despite such advances in the diagnosis of HCC, the survival rate remains low after partial hepatectomy [3–6] due to the presence of advanced liver cirrhosis or to the recurrence of HCC in the remnant liver.

We have treated patients with HCCs, mainly small HCCs, with percutaneous ethanol injection therapy [7–10]. This treatment is widely accepted for its effi-

Address for correspondence: M. Tanaka, Second Department of Internal Medicine, Kurume University School of Medicine, 67 Asahi-machi, Kurume 830, Japan. Tel.: +81-942-35-3311. Fax: +81-942-34-2623.

cacy and low incidence of complications [11,12]. This retrospective study was designed to evaluate the effects of this treatment on survival rate, and to identify the variables that significantly affected the long-term survival of the patients using Cox's multivariate analysis and the stepwise method.

Patients and Methods

Patients

Between April 1, 1984 and December 28, 1993, a total of 349 patients (239 men and 110 women) with small (<3 cm) lesions of HCC received ethanol injections as their initial therapy at Kurume University Hospital. The final diagnosis of HCC was confirmed by tumor biopsy in all patients. Their mean age was 61.8 ± 8.1 years; 171 patients were under the age of 62, and 178 patients were age 62 or older. The severity of liver dysfunction was classified as Child's A in 93 patients, Child's B in 204 patients, and Child's C in 52 patients. HBsAg was positive in 32 patients and negative in 317 patients. Serum AFP level was below 20 ng/ml in 78 patients, and 20 ng/ml or higher in 271 patients; the range was 2.9–7,500 ng/ml with a mean level of 143 ± 554.8 ng/ml. Tumors measured 20 mm or smaller in 271 patients and between 21–30 mm in 78 patients; the mean tumor size was 16.3 ± 5.8 mm. A total of 221 patients had a single tumor and 128 patients had two or three tumors. Tumor histology revealed well-differentiated HCC by biopsy in 175 patients and moderately or poorly differentiated HCC in 174 patients. When more than one HCC nodule was present, we used the histology of the largest tumor for this evaluation. Regular follow-up in 282 patients consisted of US of the liver performed at least once every 3 months at our hospital (Table 1). Sixty-seven patients were not followed regularly because they lived remote from Kurume and/or were difficult to follow for other reasons. Patients who lived remote from Kurume were contacted by telephone about their status. The period of observation ended on December 28, 1994. The mean period of observation was 1,112.2 ± 621.4 days, range 76 to 3,034 days. When lesions occupying the hepatic space were indicated to be HCC by periodic US, we performed dynamic CT scans and/or magnetic resonance imaging (MRI) in trying to detect the recurrence of HCC at an early stage. When a recurrence was diagnosed by these imaging techniques or by additional tumor biopsies, patients received ethanol injection as well as such treatments as transcatheter arterial embolization (TAE) [13,14] and regional chemotherapy using totally implanted port system [15–17] as required.

Methods

Ten clinicopathologic variables were selected for evaluation as follows: sex, age, HBsAg, (maximal) size of tumor, number of tumors, histology of tumors, serum glutamate oxaloacetic transaminase (GOT) level, Child's classification, serum

Table 1. Characteristics of patients with small HCC.

Prognostic variables	n = 349
Sex	
Men	239
Women	110
Age	
under 62	171
over 63	178
HBs-Ag[a]	
positive	32
negative	317
Child's classification	
A	93
B	204
C	52
Serum AFP[b] levels	
20 ng/ml or lower	78
21 ng/ml or higher	271
Tumor size	
20 mm or smaller	271
21 mm or larger	78
Number of tumor nodules	
solitary	221
multiple	128
Tumor histology	
well-differentiated HCC	175
moderately to poorly differentiated HCC	174
Regular follow-up	
done	282
not done	67

[a]HBs-Ag: hepatitis B surface antigen; [b]α-fetoprotein.

level of α-fetoprotein and regular follow-up after initial treatment of HCC. The significance of the prognostic value of each variable was estimated with Cox's multivariate proportional hazard model. Variables with $p < 0.05$ were selected in the stepwise method. The survival rate of the patients in relationship to each variable selected by the stepwise method was calculated by the Kaplan-Meier method.

Statistical analysis

Data are reported (mean ± SD) as statistical analyses using the Macintosh computer and the Stat View II program. The statistical significance of differences in the cumulative survival rate was analyzed by the log-rank test. A level of $p < 0.05$ was considered statistically significant.

Results

Significant prognostic variables after ethanol injection therapy

We found that sex, age, (maximal) tumor size, tumor histology, Child's classification and regular follow-up after ethanol injection were significantly related to prognosis (Table 2) using Cox's multivariate proportional hazard model (stepwise method).

Survival rate

The cumulative survival rate (Kaplan-Meier method) showed 3-year, 5-year and 7-year survival rate of 73.5%, 47.0%, and 27.0%, respectively (Table 3). Significant differences in survival rate were observed among the groups stratified by each variable, except for sex, using Cox's multivariate proportional hazard model. Survival rates differed significantly among groups stratified by tumor histology (Fig. 1) and by regular follow-up after ethanol injection therapy (Fig. 2). Child's classification was also a significant prognostic variable after ethanol injection therapy, with survival rates differing significantly between patients with Child's A and Child's C classification (Fig. 3).

Discussion

The prognosis of 349 patients with small HCC who were treated initially with ethanol injection was evaluated to determine the efficacy of this treatment. Analysis of cumulative survival rate showed a 3-year, 5-year and 7-year survival of 73.5%, 47.0% and 27.0%, respectively. Shiina et al. reported a 3-year, 5-year and 7-year survival rate of 65.0%, 44.0% and 36.0%, respectively, in 158 patients with small HCC (up to three lesions less than 3 cm in diameter) who received ethanol injection [11]. Ebara et al. reported a 3-year and 5-year survival rate of

Table 2. Significant prognostic variables for 349 patients with small hepatocellular carcinoma treated intially with ethanol injection therapy as determined by the Cox's multivariate proportional hazard model.

	Coefficient	p value	Relative risk	95% confidence interval
Sex	0.836	0.0003	2.307	(1.462-3.639)
Age	0.559	0.0031	1.749	(1.208-2.534)
Tumor size	0.471	0.0182	1.601	(1.083-2.366)
Tumor histology	0.825	<0.0001	2.283	(1.524-3.420)
Child's classification				
Child A vs. B	0.893	0.0015	2.442	(1.409-4.230)
Child B vs. C	0.567	0.0148	1.763	(1.117-2.783)
Regular follow-up	1.056	<0.0001	2.874	(1.961-4.210)

Table 3. Cumulative survival rate of patients with small hepatocellular carcinoma stratified by each variable.

Variables	3-year survival (%)	5-year survival (%)	7-year survival (%)	p value
Sex				p = 0.0751
men (n = 239)	71.2	42.5	23.9	
women (n = 110)	77.8	56.9	37.4	
Age				p = 0.0137
under 62 (n = 171)	80.7	51.9	29.0	
over 63 (n = 178)	64.5	38.8	23.7	
Child's classification				p = 0.0006
Child A (n = 93)	87.3	61.2	28.8	p = 0.0368 (A vs. B)
Child B (n = 204)	73.9	43.7	26.6	p = 0.0145 (B vs. C)
Child C (n = 52)	49.8	34.2	0.0	
Tumor histology				p < 0.0001
well-differentiated HCC[a] (n = 175)	84.0	62.7	36.7	
moderate to poorly differentiated HCC[a] (n = 174)	63.2	31.8	19.0	
Tumor size				p = 0.0002
20 mm or smaller (n = 271)	79.0	56.4	26.9	
21 mm or larger (n = 78)	54.5	29.4	16.8	
Regular follow-up				p < 0.0001
done (n = 282)	81.2	53.9	31.7	
not done (n = 67)	43.9	18.5	12.4	
Total cases (n = 349)	73.5	47.0	27.0	

[a]HCC: hepatocellular carcinoma.

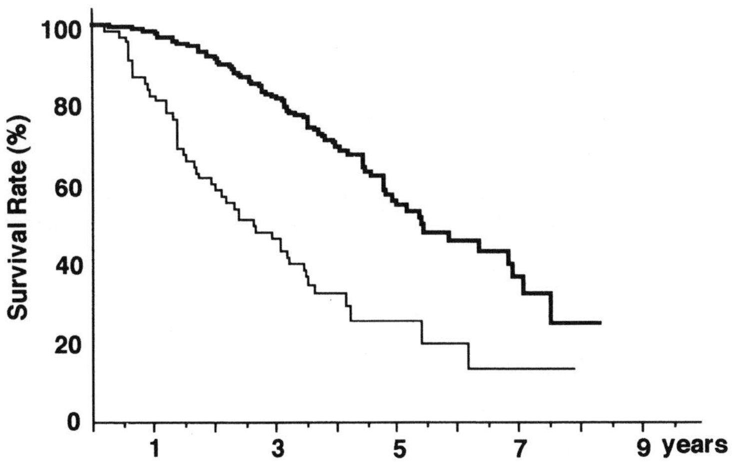

Fig. 1. Relationship between cumulative survival rate and tumor histology in patients with small HCC treated initially with percutaneous ethanol injection therapy. The group with well-differentiated HCC (n = 175) is represented by the thick line; the group with moderately to poorly differentiated HCC (n = 174) is represented by the thin line.

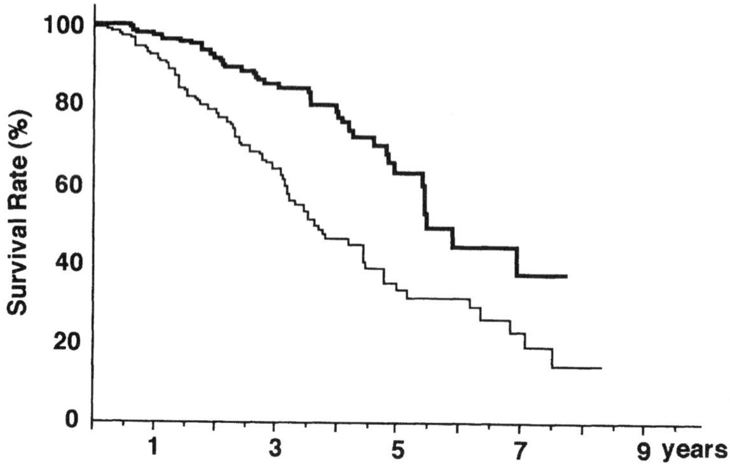

Fig. 2. Relationship between cumulative survival rate and regular follow-up in patients with small HCC treated initially with ethanol injection therapy. The group with regular follow-up (n = 282) is represented by the thick line and the group without regular follow-up (n = 67) is represented by the thin line.

62.0% and 28.0%, respectively, in 95 patients with small HCC [10]. Lencioni et al. reported a 3-year and 5-year survival rate of 68.0% and 32.0%, respectively, in 105 western patients with HCC (up to four lesions less than 5 cm in diameter) [12]. Our findings are consistent with those results. We compared the results of our treatment with ethanol injection with the results obtained with hepatectomy

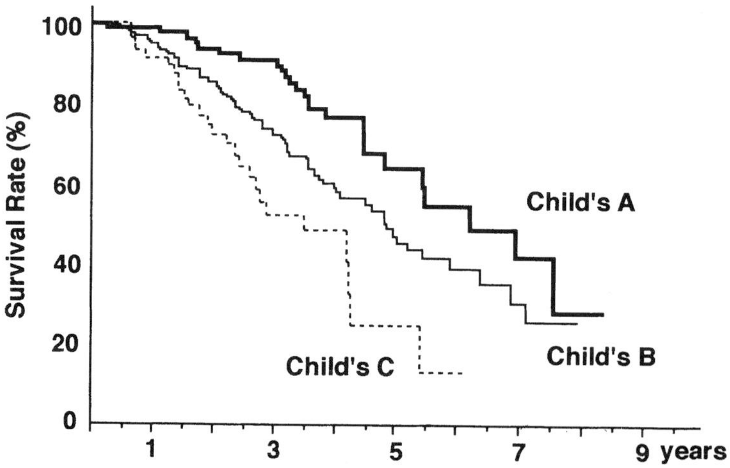

Fig. 3. Relationship between cumulative survival rate and Child's classification in patients with small HCC treated initially with ethanol injection therapy. Child's A group (n = 93) is represented by the thick solid line; Child's B group (n = 204) is represented by the thin solid line; Child's C group (n = 52) is represented by the dotted line.

for patients with similar background. The 5-year survival rate of 3,225 patients with small HCC (up to three lesions 1–3 cm in diameter) who underwent hepatectomy was 60.0% at clinical stage I (categorized by Liver Cancer Study Group of Japan [18] as ascites absent, serum total bilirubin < 2.0 mg/dl serum albumin > 3.5 g/dl, indocyanine green retention rate at 15 min < 15% prothrombin time > 80%), and 43.3% at clinical stage II (ascites disappeared with treatment, 2.0 mg/dl < total bilirubin < 3.0 mg/dl, 3.0 g/dl < serum albumin < 3.5 g/dl, 15% < indocyanine green retention rate at 15 min < 40%, 50% < prothrombin time < 80%) [19]. The survival rate in our study was 63.7% for patients in clinical stage I, and 44.5% for patients in clinical stage II (data not shown). Overall, the patients treated with ethanol injection survived as long as those treated surgically. Due to the low incidence of complications and the fact that patients did not require intensive care after treatment, repeated injections of ethanol were safely administered in cases of recurrence. Ethanol injection therapy thus may be selected for the initial treatment for patients with small HCC. We then evaluated the significance of prognostic variables for patients with small HCC. Cox's multivariate analysis revealed the significant variables to be age, Child's classification, tumor histology, tumor size and regular follow-up. The difference in survival rates was highly significant among groups stratified by tumor histology and regular follow-up. Tumor size was one of the most significant prognostic variables in this study. HCC originated as well-differentiated tumors and become less differentiated as the size of the tumor increased [20]. The initial treatment with ethanol injection of patients with moderately to poorly differentiated HCC detected by US did not necessarily prevent the occurrence of intrahepatic metastasis, even when the maximal size of the tumor was < 3 cm. A poor prognosis was demonstrated in such patients. Survival rates did not differ significantly among groups stratified by number of tumors, indicating that periodic US may have detected HCCs at an early stage, and that the tumors may have been completely necrotized by the injection of ethanol. Thus, the number of tumors present did not greatly influence the duration of survival after the administration of ethanol in patients with HCC who were followed regularly. We performed regular follow-up at least once every 3 months in most cases, except with 67 patients. In cases of tumor recurrence with moderate to poor differentiation and in which periodic US had not been performed, it was difficult to achieve a local cure by ethanol injection. Patients with a high risk of recurrence were informed of the necessity for regular follow-up. Many of the HCC patients were HCV antibody-positive, so it is not surprising that older patients in whom HCC had occurred 25 to 30 years after the initial HCV infection [21] showed a high incidence of carcinoma and a poor prognosis. The incidence of extrahepatic disorders such as heart disease increased with age, and presumably also influenced the survival rate of patients with HCC. The survival rate of patients with Child's C classification was lower than that of Child's A classification. Our results indicate that the prognosis following ethanol injection treatment of HCC may depend on the severity of liver dysfunction. Regular follow-up as well as the differentiation of hepatocellular carcinoma contributed to an improved survival rate of patients with small HCC following the percutaneous administration of ethanol.

References

1. Kitamura S, Ishii H, Tatsuya M, Ishikawa H, Hiyama T, Tsukuma H, Kasugai H, Tanaka S, Kitamura T, Ishiguro S. Liver with hypoechoic nodular pattern as a risk factor for hepatocellular carcinoma. Gastroenterology 1995;108:1778–1784.
2. Kondo F, Wada K, Nagato Y, Nakajima T, Kondo Y, Hirooka N, Ebara M, Ohto M, Okuda K. Biopsy diagnosis of well-differentiated hepatocellular carcinoma based on new morphologic criteria. Hepatology 1989;9:751–755.
3. Takayasu K, Muramatsu Y, Moriyama N, Hasegawa H, Makuuchi N, Okazaki N, Hirohashi S, Tsugane S. Clinical and radiologic assessment of the results of hepatectomy for small hepatocellular carcinoma and therapeutic arterial embolization for postoperative recurrence. Cancer 1989;64:1848–1852.
4. Ikeda K, Saitoh S, Tsubota A, Arase Y, Chayama K, Kumada H, Watanabe G, Tsurumaru M. Risk factors for tumor recurrence and prognosis after curative resection of hepatocellular carcinoma. Cancer 1993;71:19–25.
5. Yamanaka N, Okamoto E, Toyosaka A, Mitunobu M, Fujihara S, Kato T, Fujimoto J, Oriyama T, Furukawa K, Kawamura E. Prognostic factors after hepatectomy for hepatocellular carcinomas: a univariate and multivariate analysis. Cancer 1990;65:1104–1110.
6. Nagao T, Inoue S, Yosimi F, Sodeyama M, Omori Y, Mizuta T, Kawano N, Morioka Y. Postoperative recurrence of hepatocellular carcinoma. Ann Surg 1990;211:28–33.
7. Tanikawa K, Majima Y. Percutaneous ethanol injection therapy for recurrent hepatocellular carcinoma. Hepato-Gastroenterol 1993;40:324–327.
8. Livraghi T, Festi D, Monti F, Salmi A, Vettori C. US-guided percutaneous alcohol injection of small hepatic and abdominal tumors. Radiology 1986;161:309–312.
9. Shiina S, Yasuda H, Muto H, Tagawa K, Unuma T, Ibukuro K, Inoue Y, Takanashi R. Percutaneous ethanol injection in the treatment of liver neoplasms. AJR 1987;149:949–952.
10. Ebara M, Ohto M, Sugiura N, Kita K, Yoshikawa M, Okuda K, Kondo F, Kondo Y. Percutaneous ethanol injection for the treatment of small hepatocellular carcinoma. Study of 95 patients. J Gastroenterol Hepatol 1990;5:616–626.
11. Shiina S, Imamur M, Nishimura S, Ogura K, Okamoto M, Tanaka T, Kato N, Niwa Y, Shiratori Y, Omata M. Percutaneous ethanol injection therapy (PEIT) for small hepatocellular carcinoma. Syoukakika 1994;19:120–128. (In Japanese)
12. Lencioni R, Bartolozzi C, Caramella D, Paolicchi A, Carrai M, Maltinti G, Capria A, Tafi A, Conte PF, Bevilacqua G. Treatment of small hepatocellular carcinoma with percutaneous ethanol injection. Analysis of prognostic factors in 105 western patients. Cancer 1995;76:1737–1746.
13. Yamada R, Sato M, Kawabata M, Nakatsuka H, Nakamura K, Takashima S. Hepatic artery embolization in 120 patients with unresectable hepatoma. Radiology 1983;148:397–401.
14. Bronowicki JP, Vetter D, Dumas F, Boudjema K, Bader R, Weiss AM, Wenger JJ, Boissel P, Bigard MA, Doffoel M. Transcatheter oily chemoembolization for hepatocellular carcinoma. Cancer 1994;74:16–24.
15. Nakamura K, Takashima S, Takada K, Fujimoto K, Kaminou T, Nakatsuka H, Minakuchi K, Onoyama Y. Clinical evaluation of intermittent arterial infusion chemotherapy with an implanted reservoir for hepatocellular carcinoma. Cancer Chemother Pharmacol 1992;31:93–98.
16. Yodono H, Takekawa S, Tarusawa K, Ikami I, Kanehira J, Saito Y, Takahashi S, Sasaki T, Nishi N, Kimura T, Oikawa S, Shibutani K, Shinohara A, Anbai A, Sasaki R, Sasaki Y, Noda H. Combination therapy consist of arterial infusion chemotherapy (EPF, EAP) and transcatheter arterial embolization (TAE). Cancer Chemother Pharmacol 1994;33:79–83.

17. Yoshikawa M, Saosho H, Ebara M, Iijima T, Iwama S, Endo F, Kimura M, Shimamura Y, Suzuki Y, Nakano T, Fukuyama Y, Fujise K, Nambu M, Ohto M. A randomized trial of intrahepatic arterial infusion of 4′-epidoxorubicin with lipiodol versus 4′-epidoxorubicin alone in the treatment of hepatocellular carcinoma. Cancer Chemother Pharmacol 1994;33:149–152.
18. Liver Cancer Study Group of Japan. The general rules for the clinical and pathological study of primary liver cancer. Jpn J Surg 1989;19:198–129.
19. Ryu M, Shimamura Y, Kawano N, Iwasaki M, Kinoshita T, Konishi M, Furuse J, Yoshino M. The present condition of the treatment for HCC. Syoukakigeka 1995;18:415–419. (In Japanese)
20. Kenmochi K, Sugihara S, Kojiro M. Relationship of histologic grade of hepatocellular carcinoma (HCC) to tumor size, and demonstration of tumor cells of multiple different grades in single HCC. Liver 1987;7:18–26.
21. Kiyosawa K, Sodeyama T, Tanaka E, Gibo Y, Yoshizawa K, Nakano Y, Furuta S, Akahane Y, Nishioka K, Purcell RH, Alter HJ. Interrelationship of blood transfusion, non-A, non-B hepatitis and hepatocellular carcinoma: analysis of antibody to hepatitis C virus. Hepatology 1990; 12:671–675.

Progress in Hepatology, Volume 3.
Hepatocellular Carcinoma.
M. Yamanaka, G. Toda and T. Tanaka, editors.

Efficacy of percutaneous acetic acid injection for small hepatocellular carcinoma

Kunihiko Ohnishi
Third Department of Medicine, Saitama Medical School, Saitama, Japan

Abstract. To assess the efficacy of ultrasound (US)-guided percutaneous acetic acid injection (PAI) for small hepatocellular carcinomas (HCCs) for long-term prognosis, PAI using 15 to 50% acetic acid was performed in 99 patients with one to four HCCs smaller than 3 cm during the past 7.5 years. During the series of treatment sessions for each patient, the same concentration of acetic acid was used. All tumors could be treated successfully with PAI. The number of treatment sessions for similar tumor size were less when the higher concentrations of acetic acid were used. No serious complications occurred. The 1-, 3- and 5-year survival rates were 98, 81 and 54%, respectively. To assess the efficacy of PAI using 50% acetic acid for small HCCs in comparison to percutaneous ethanol injection (PEI), the randomized controlled study was prospectively performed in 60 patients with small HCCs. The local recurrence rate was significantly lower with PAI than with PEI. The survival rate was significantly higher in PAI than in PEI. In conclusion: PAI using 15 to 50% acetic acid is an effective therapy for small HCC for long-term prognosis. PAI using 50% acetic acid is superior to PEI in the treatment of small HCCs.

Keywords: hepatocellular carcinoma (HCC), local recurrence rate, percutaneous ethanol injection (PEI), percutaneous acetic acid injection (PAI), small hepatocellular carcinoma, survival rate, ultrasonography.

Introduction

Hepatocellular carcinoma (HCC) is one of the major human malignancies with poor prognosis in eastern Asia as well as sub-Saharan Africa [1]; an estimated incidence could be evaluated as 1,250,000 deaths per year worldwide [2].

Early detection plans for HCC are expected to increase the number of small HCCs detected for surgical resection in endemic regions [3,4]. The survival data reported by surgical group after HCC resection have been improving over the last decade, mainly because of ever-smaller sizes of the resected neoplasms [3—5]. Some groups have thus achieved 50% 5-year survival in patients with small, asymptomatic HCCs [4]. Orthotopic liver transplantation (OLT) has been proved to be an effective treatment for small, unresectable HCCs in patients with cirrhosis [5,6]. However, surgical resection or OLT is possible in a much smaller proportion of cases because of impairment of liver function due to underlying liver cirrhosis or due to very few donors for transplantation.

This has prompted the development of other potentially curative therapeutic

Address for correspondence: Kunihiko Ohnishi MD, Third Department of Medicine, Saitama Medical School, 38 Morohongo-cho, Moroyama-cho, Iruma-gun, Saitama 350-04, Japan.

modalities such as transcatheter hepatic arterial embolization (TAE) [7] and ultrasound (US)-guided percutaneous injection of materials to kill cancer cells [8–15]. The latter can be indicated for both hypervascular and hypovascular HCCs while TAE is effective for only hypervascular HCCs but not hypovascular HCCs, the incidence of which is high among small HCCs. The effect of percutaneous ethanol injection (PEI) on prognosis has been reported to be almost comparable to surgical resection [4,9–12], although a large number of treatment sessions are required [8–13] and recurrence of primary lesion is relatively high [10–14]. In the course of development of US guided percutaneous injection of a material to kill cancer cells, we took up acetic acid that has a strong ability to penetrate cells with a capability of dissolving lipids and extracting collagen [16,17].

At first, we demonstrated in rats that the capability of acetic acid to necrotize hepatocytes increased with an increase of its concentrations until its killing effect plateaued at 50% and that its capability at 15% was equal to or greater than the capability of absolute alcohol to necrotize hepatocytes [18,19]. Based on these results, we developed a US-guided method called percutaneous acetic acid injection (PAI), using a 15, 20, 30, 40 and 50% acetic acid solution [18–20] and we reported that PAI using 15 to 50% acetic acid became an effective therapy for small HCCs. Recently, we reported that PAI using 50% acetic acid was superior to segmental TAE in hypervascular small HCC because both survival rate and cancer-free survival rate were significantly higher in the former than in the latter [21].

In this article, we report the results of PAI for small HCCs for long-term prognosis and of the randomized controlled study of PAI and PEI for small HCCs.

Methods

Ninety-nine patients with one to four HCCs smaller than 3 cm in diameter were treated by PAI using concentrations of 15, 20, 30, 40 and 50% acetic acid during the period from May 1988 to September 1995.

Clinical characteristics of the groups treated by different concentrations of acetic acid are shown in Table 1. All patients were classified on admission according to Child's grade for portal hypertension [22]; for Child C, a single worst criterion was used (albumin $\leqslant 3$ mg/dl, total bilirubin $\geqslant 3$ mg/dl, massive ascites or hepatic encephalopathy). The two-dimensional size of tumor was assessed from the US image. The large or largest tumor was called the main tumor if the patient had two to four tumors. If the patient had only one tumor, it was called the main tumor. Diagnosis of HCC was made by biopsy using a 18- or 21-gauge needle (Hirata Sangyo Co., Tokyo, Japan) under US guidance. The baseline data used were (a) US findings and measurement of two-dimensional size of tumor, (b) serum alpha-fetoprotein (AFP) levels, (c) plasma PIVKA-II levels, (d) angiographic findings and (e) computed tomographic (CT) findings with plain scans and helical dynamic as well as contrast-enhanced scans

Table 1. Clinical characteristics of each acetic acid group.

	Acetic acid concentrations (%)				
	15	20	30	40	50
No. of patient	20	11	3	14	51
Child class					
A	15 (75)	8 (73)	2 (67)	11 (79)	33 (65)
B	0	0	1 (33)	1 (7)	3 (6)
C	5 (25)	3 (27)	0	2 (14)	15 (29)
Diameter of main tumor					
1—2 cm	15 (75)	8 (73)	3 (100)	9 (64)	32 (63)
2—3 cm	5 (25)	3 (27)	0	5 (36)	19 (37)
No. of tumor					
1	16 (80)	10 (91)	0	9 (64)	44 (86)
2—4	4 (20)	1 (9)	3 (100)	5 (36)	7 (14)

Note: Number in parentheses indicates the percentage in each item. There was no significant difference in each item among each acetic acid group.

after bolus administration of contrast material. CT examinations were performed as described previously [20] or with commercially available helical CT scanners (X-vision, Toshiba Medical, Tokyo, Japan) by using a 1.5-s gantry rotation period, 120 kV and 165 mA. An unenhanced conventional scan was initially obtained by using 10-mm sections every 10 mm through the entire liver to serve as a baseline study for attenuation measurements. Then, the patients received 120 ml iohexol (Omnipaque, 300 mg/ml; Daiichi, Tokyo, Japan) biphasically; with first 75 ml iohexol administered at a rate of 5 ml/s and 45 ml iohexol administered at 3 ml/s. Helical scanning was begun 20—25 s after the initiation of injection of iohexol at the diaphragm and proceeded caudally. Imaging parameters included section thickness, 10 mm; table increment speed 15 mm/s; axial images constructed every 10 mm; scanning duration, 20 s. After helical scanning the patients received 70 ml of iohexol again at a rate of 1 ml/s and a delayed conventional scan was obtained 180 s after the initial injection of iohexol by using 10 mm sections every 10 mm through the entire liver.

The instruments and procedure for PAI are shown in Fig. 1. The procedure for PAI was as follows. After local anesthesia using 0.5 or 1.0% xylocaine at the site of puncture, a thin needle (outer diameter 22-gauge, length 15 or 20 cm) with marks for every 1 cm and rubber stopper (Hatsuko Co., Tokyo, Japan) was introduced percutaneously into the tumor under US guidance using a linear, convex, or sector puncture probe (Aloka, Tokyo, Japan) for real-time US. The stylet was withdrawn and the needle was connected to a syringe filled with 15 to 50% acetic acid solution via an extension tube (Terumo Co., Tokyo, Japan). Acetic acid was slowly injected until the echogenic area appearing immediately after injection covered the entire tumor, or a strong resistance to the injection pressure was felt. The amount injected was approximately 1—3 ml for 1- to 2-cm HCCs and

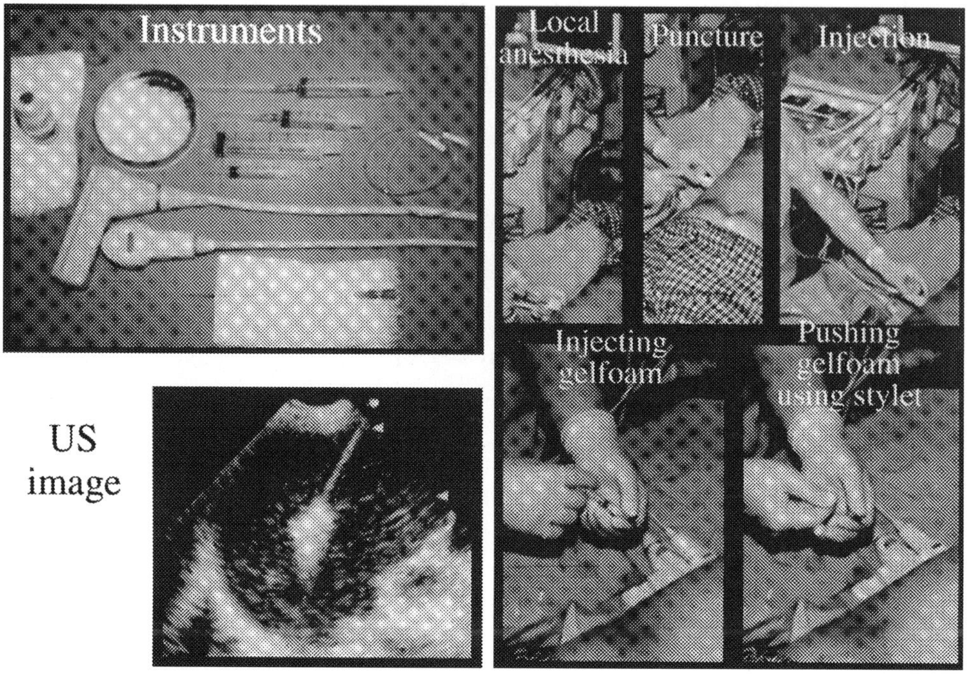

Fig. 1. Instruments and procedures for PAI and PEI.

approximately 2–5 ml for 2- to 3-cm HCCs. Then, the needle was withdrawn slowly while a mixture of Gelfoam (Upjohn, Kalamazoo, MI, USA) powder and saline was pushed by the stylet into the puncture hole in the liver parenchyma to prevent local pain caused by leakage of acetic acid or ethanol. It would also prevent backflow of tumor content which could cause dissemination of cancer cells into the surrounding tissue. One injection was given in each treatment session. PAI treatment session was performed twice a week and repeated until the tumor changed to a very hyperechoic mass as a whole on US or a crescent-shaped very hyperechoic mass (Fig. 2). During a series of treatment sessions for one patient, the same concentration of acetic acid was used. To assess the adequacy of PAI, tumor biopsy using 21-gauge needle, plain, helical dynamic and contrast-enhanced CT and angiography were performed again within two weeks after the last treatment session. If no viable cancer cells were found in the biopsy specimen, the lesion changed to hypoattenuating on helical dynamic and contrast-enhanced CT, and there was neither hypervascularity nor staining of the lesion on angiography, then PAI was discontinued. If viable tumor cells were found or the lesion had hyperattenuating areas or hypervascularity or staining, PAI was continued for one or two more sessions, followed by another biopsy using 21-gauge needle, CT and angiography.

From August 1993 to September 1995, 60 patients with one to four HCCs smaller than 3 cm, entered a randomized controlled trial aimed at investigating

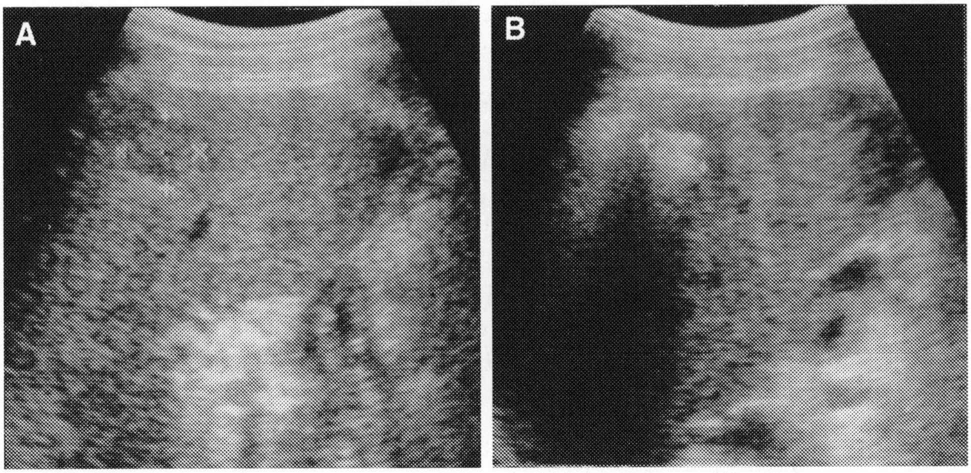

Fig. 2. Ultrasound changes of small HCC after PAI. A hypoechoic (19 × 17 mm) tumor (A) changed to a very hyperechoic tumor as a whole (B) immediately after the third session of PAI.

the efficacy and safety of PAI in comparison with PEI in the treatment of small HCC after a written informed consent was obtained from each patient and family member(s). They were randomly allocated by sealed envelop to the PAI group (n = 31) or the PEI group (n = 29). Both PAI and PEI were performed on in-patient basis. PAI and PEI were performed as described above. In brief, PAI using 50% acetic acid solution or PEI using absolute ethanol was performed twice a week and repeated until the total amount of absolute ethanol (V1) or 50% acetic acid (V2) injected for all sessions to treat each tumor reached the volume calculated using the equation 1 proposed by Shiina et al. [10] and the equation 2 made by us, considering that a capability of 50% acetic acid to necrotize hepatocytes is more than 3 times that of absolute ethanol [18,19]: equation 1, V1 (ml) = 4/3 × 3.14 × (r + 0.5)3; equation 2, V2 (ml) = 4/3 × 3.14 × (r + 0.5)3 × 1/3; r (cm) = radius of each tumor. The assessment of adequacy of PAI or PEI was performed as described above. Posttreatment follow-up included US scan every 3 months, measurement of serum AFP and plasma PIVKA-II levels every month and CT every 6 months. Side effects of PAI were assessed from changes in symptoms and signs as well as hematological and biochemical findings.

Statistical analysis

Results are given as mean ± SD. Comparisons were made by the Student's t test and χ^2 test. Cumulative survival rate, rate of local recurrence (re-enlargement of the original HCC), and cancer-free survival rate were calculated from the time of diagnosis of the original HCC by the Kaplan-Meier method [23]. Statistical analysis was made by the log-rank test [24]. Values of $p < 0.05$ were considered significant.

Results

Relationship among tumor size, acetic acid concentration injected and number of treatment sessions.

All tumors could be treated successfully with PAI despite the differences in acetic acid concentrations. The number of treatment sessions to adequately control 1- to 2-cm HCCs was 3.4±1.4, 3.2±1.3, 3.3±1.5, 2.6±1.0, 2.1±0.9 in PAI using 15, 20, 30, 40, 50%, respectively ($p<0.001$ between 50 and 15% acetic acid groups, $p<0.005$ between 40 and 15% acetic acid groups), and that of control 2- and 3-cm HCCs was less in the order of 15, 20, 40 and 50% acetic acid groups (5.0±1.9, 4.7±0.6, 4.3±0.8, 2.9±0.6) ($p<0.005$ between 50 and 15% acetic acid group).

Effect of PAI on tumor

The effect of PAI on tumor was examined histologically. Biopsy specimens obtained shortly after the last treatment showed coagulation necrosis and fibrosis of various degrees in all. Twenty patients underwent aspiration of the tumor with a thin needle within a week after the last treatment session. A small amount of brownish fluid was drawn from the tumor, which is suggestive of partial liquefaction of the necrotic tissue (Fig. 3). Amino acid analysis was performed using high performance liquid chromatography in these brownish fluids of four

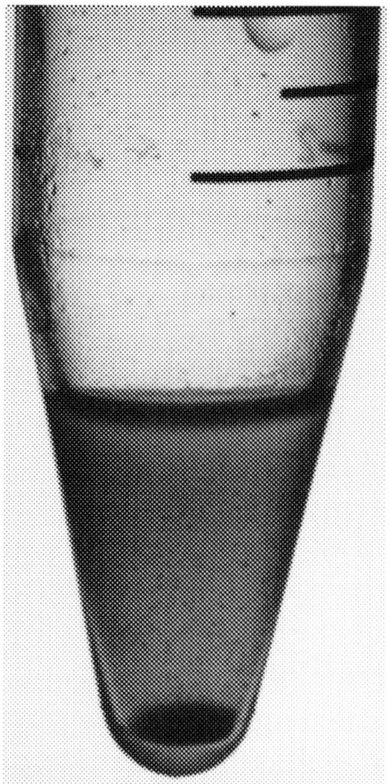

Fig. 3. Brownish fluid drawn from the tumor after PAI.

patients. High concentrations of hydroxylysine (22 ~ 155 nmol/ml) and lysine (479 ~ 3,500 nmol/ml) were detected.

Tumor recurrence

Only three (2.4%) of 124 primary HCCs treated with PAI showed local recurrence. However, a new HCC occurred frequently elsewhere in the liver. Thus, 1-, 2-, 3-, 4- and 5-year recurrence rate for HCCs were 14, 39, 46, 54 and 63%, respectively.

Causes of death, survival rate and cancer-free survival rate

Thirty-two of 99 patients died: the cause of death were hepatic failure in 41%, HCC in 31% and others. The 1-, 2-, 3-, 4-, 5-, 6- and 7-year survival rates of all 99 patients were 96, 86, 81, 67, 54, 46 and 35%, respectively. The 1-, 2-, 3-, 4-, 5-, 6- and 7-year cancer-free survival rates were 83, 56, 50, 36, 29, 29 and 29%, respectively. With respect to the size of main tumors, the 1-, 2-, 3-, 4- and 5-year survival rates were 96, 93, 93, 81 and 73%, respectively, in patients with 1- to 1.5-cm HCCs, 100, 90, 90, 74 and 54% in patients with 1.5- to 2-cm HCCs, and 91, 75, 57, 44 and 44% in patients with 2- to 3-cm HCCs ($p < 0.001$). With respect to the number of lesions, there was no significant difference of survival rate between patients with a single tumor and patients with two to four tumors (data not shown). With respect to the hepatic functional reserve, the 1-, 2-, 3-, 4- and 5-year survival rates were 99, 93, 89, 77 and 62%, respectively, in Child A+B patients and 88, 66, 59, 37 and 37 in Child C patients ($p < 0.001$). With respect to the acetic acid concentrations, the survival rate was in an increasing order of 15, 20, 30, 40 and 50% acetic acid groups (Fig. 4) although there was

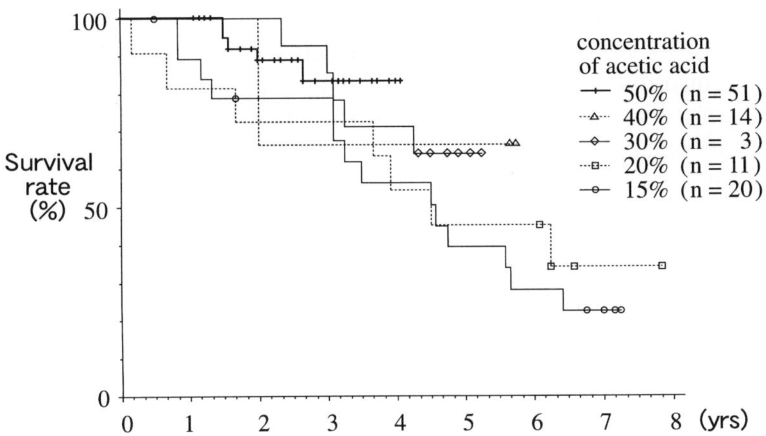

Fig. 4. Survival rates for 99 patients with one to four HCCs smaller than 3 cm treated with PAI in relation to acetic acid concentration.

no significant difference in size of main tumor, number of tumors and Child class among each group (Table 1).

Comparison of PAI and PEI

PAI and PEI groups did not show any significant differences in age (63±9 years vs. 63±12 years), male/female ratio (20/11 vs. 19/10), Child class: A/B/C ratio (21/2/8 vs. 16/7/6), C-viral liver cirrhosis/others ratio (26/5 vs. 23/6), size of tumor (1.8±0.5 cm vs. 1.9±0.6 cm) and number of tumor: 1/2—4 (26/5 vs. 25/4). The number of treatment sessions (2.5±0.9 vs. 3.9±1.6, $p<0.001$) were significantly less in tumors treated with PAI than those treated with PEI. All original tumors could be treated successfully by either PAI or PEI. However, 8% of tumors treated with PAI and 37% of tumors treated with PEI showed local recurrence (re-enlargement of the original HCC) ($p<0.01$). In addition, a new HCC occurred elsewhere in the liver in 39% of PAI group patients and 52% of PEI group patient (not significant). Three PAI group patients died: the causes of death were HCC in one patient, hepatic failure in one patient, and variceal bleeding in the other. In contrast, 11 PEI group patients died: the causes of death were HCC in four patients, hepatic failure in four patients, variceal bleeding in two patients, and suicide in one patient. The 1- and 2-year survival rates were 100 and 94%, respectively in PAI group and 81 and 63% in PEI group ($p = 0.0137$). No serious complications that necessitated intensive care were encountered during and after either PAI or PEI therapy. After injection of acetic acid or absolute ethanol, most patients complained of transient pain and showed a mild or moderate elevation of body temperature, which returned to normal within 3 days.

Discussion

The present study demonstrated several issues:

PAI therapy using 15 to 50% acetic acid was very effective for HCCs smaller than 3 cm in long-term prognosis, and the use of 50% acetic acid would be preferable to lower concentrations because it reduced the number of treatment sessions and tended to increase the survival rate.

The number of treatment sessions for small HCC were significantly less in PAI using 50% acetic acid compared with PEI. The presence of fibrous capsule and fibrous septa within the mass is one of the gross characteristics of HCC in the Far East [25]. The frequency of capsule and septum formation runs parallel with an increase of tumor size [26]. The fibrous capsule seems to be formed primarily by the condensation of fibrous components in the adjacent liver parenchyma due to compression which follows the expansion of the tumor. In septum formation, two mechanisms have been suggested: 1) the entangled old capsule within the cancerous tissue following extracapsular tumor growth becomes septa, or 2) the fine fibrous bands formed at the boundary of the cancerous tissue with different histologic features become the septa [26]. The fibrous capsule consists of at least type I and type III collagens. Type IV collagens were localized around the vessels in the fibrous capsule [27]. Thus, to treat small HCC of 1 to 3 cm successfully with PEI, one needs at least as many treatment sessions as the same number of nodules formed by septa within the same mass, because ethanol injected into one tumor nodule cannot penetrate the septa. In contrast, less injection sessions are required in PAI because acetic acid injected into one nodule will penetrate through septa largely because of its low pH, which induces swelling of the fibers and promotes the dissociation of intramolecular cross-links containing aldimine bonds of collagen [16,17] in the septa as suggested in the present study.

The local recurrence rate was significantly lower in tumors treated with PAI compared with PEI, reflecting the said property of acetic acid [16,17]. We have already reported that the liver specimen resected after PAI showed complete necrosis of intracapsular metastatic foci as well as of main encapsulated tumor [20].

Recurrence of new HCC(s), different from the original tumor occurred just as frequently in the liver after PAI and PEI. Such recurrence was perhaps related to multiple metachronous or unnoticed, synchronous tumors or intrahepatic metastatic tumors not detected even with the latest liver imaging techniques [28,29]. However, the possibility still exists, even if it is rare that insertion of thin needle into HCCs and the tumor biopsy using a 18- or 21-gauge needle expedited migration of cancer cells. Alternatively, the entire liver is cirrhotic and probably contains innumerable regenerative nodules. Therefore, the entire remaining liver is predisposed to the development of multiple HCCs [30].

The survival rate was significantly better with PAI than with PEI. This is perhaps attributed, at least in part, to the lower local recurrence rate. Significant complications (portal vein thrombosis, cholangitis, intraperitoneal hemorrhage), reported with PEI by others [19,10,12], did not occur after either method in the present study. The lack of complication may be related to our technique of sealing the puncture hole with Gelfoam powder which is not done in PEI by others [8–14].

Conclusion

PAI using 50% acetic acid is a very effective therapy for small HCCs for long-term prognosis, it is superior to PEI, and it entails less burden for the patient as well as less load for the physician.

References

1. Okuda K, Okuda H. Primary liver cell carcinoma. In: McIntyre N, Benhamou J-P, Bircher J, Rizzetto M, Rodes J (eds) Oxford Textbook of Clinical Hepatology. Vol. 2. Oxford, England: Oxford University Press, 1991:1019–1052.
2. Fong Y, Blumgart LH, Cohen AM. Surgical treatment of colorectal metastases to the liver. CA Cancer J Clin 1995;45:50–62.
3. Ohnishi K, Tanabe Y, Ryu M, Isono K, Yamamoto Y, Usui S, Iwama S, Sugita S, Nomura F, Oku-

da K. Prognosis of hepatocellular carcinoma smaller than 5 cm in relation to treatment: study of 100 patients. Hepatology 1987;7:1285–1290.

4. Makuuchi M, Kosuge T, Takayama T, Yamazaki S, Kakazu T, Miyagawa S, Kawasaki S. Surgery for small liver cancers. Semin Surg Oncol 1993;9:298–304.
5. Iwatsuki S, Starzl TE, Sheahan DC, Yokoyama I, Demetris AJ, Todo S, Tzakis AG, Van Tihel DH, Carr B, Selby R, Madariaga J. Hepatic resection versus transplantation for hepatocellular carcinoma. Ann Surg 1991;214:221–229.
6. Mazzaferro V, Regalia E, Doci R, Andreola S, Pulvirenti A, Bozzentti F, Ammatuna M, Morabito A, Gennari L. Liver transplantation for the treatment of small hepatocellular carcinomas in patients with cirrhosis. N Eng J Med 1996;334:693–699.
7. Matsui O, Kadoya M, Yoshikawa J, Gabata T, Arai K, Demachi H, Miyayama S, Takashima T, Unoura M, Kobayashi K. Small hepatocellular carcinoma: treatment with subsegmental transcatheter arterial embolization. Radiology 1993;188:79–83.
8. Sheu JC, Sung JL, Huang GT, Chen DS, Yang PM, Lai MY, Wei TC, Su CT, Tsang YM, Lee CZ, Chen JC, Hsu HC. Intratumor injection of absolute ethanol under ultrasound guidance for the treatment of small hepatocellular carcinoma. Hepatogastroenterology 1987;34:255–261.
9. Ebara M, Ohto M, Sugiura N, Okuda K, Kondo F, Kondo K. Percutaneous ethanol injection for the treatment of small hepatocellular carcinoma: study of 95 patients. J Gastroenterol Hepatol 1990;5:616–626.
10. Shiina S, Tagawa K, Niwa Y, Unuma T, Komatsu Y, Yoshiura K, Hamada E, Takahashi M, Shiratori Y, Terano A, Omata M, Kawauchi N, Inoue H. Percutaneous ethanol injection therapy for hepatocellular carcinoma: results in 146 patients. AJR 1993;160:1023–1028.
11. Tanikawa K, Majima Y. Percutaneous ethanol injection therapy for recurrent hepatocellular carcinoma. Hepatogastroenterology 1993;40:324–327.
12. Livraghi T, Giorgio A, Marin G, Salmi A, Siode I, Bolondi L, Pompili M, Brunello F, Lazzaroni S, Torzilli G, Zucchi A. Hepatocellular carcinoma and cirrhosis in 746 patients: long-term results of percutaneous ethanol injection. Radiology 1995;197:101–108.
13. Castells A, Bruix J, Bru C, Fuster J, Vilana R, Navasa M, Ayuso C, Boix L, Visa J, Rodes J. Treatment of small hepatocellular carcinoma in cirrhotic patients: a cohort study comparing surgical resection and percutaneous ethanol injection. Hepatology 1993;18:1121–1126.
14. Hirata M, Nishimura N. Hepatocellular carcinoma recurrence after percutaneous ethanol injection therapy: comparison of tumors with or without a septum. Jpn J Med Ultrasonics 1993;20: 548–554. (In Japanese)
15. Honda N, Guo Q, Uchida H, Ohishi H, Hiasa Y. Percutaneous hot saline injection therapy for hepatic tumors: an alternative to percutaneous ethanol injection therapy. Radiology 1994; 190:53–57.
16. Timpl R, Wiedemann H, Delden VV, Furthmayr H, Kuhn K. A network model for the organization of type IV collagen molecules in basement membranes. Eur J Biochem 1981;120:203–211.
17. Miller E, Rhodes RK. Preparation and characterization of the different types of collagen. In: Cunningham LW, Frederiksen DW (eds) Methods in Enzymology. Vol 82. Structural and Contractile Proteins. Part A. Extracellular Matrix. New York: Academic Press, 1982:23–64.
18. Ohnishi K, Chin N, Ito S. Percutaneous acetic acid injection therapy for hepatocellular carcinoma less than 3 cm in diameter. Acta Hepatol Jpn 1993;34:504–516. (in Japanese)
19. Ohnishi K, Ohyama N, Ito S, Fujiwara K. Ultrasound guided intratumor injection of acetic acid for the treatment of small hepatocellular carcinoma. Radiology 1994;193:747–752.
20. Ohnishi K, Nomura F, Ito S, Fujiwara K. Prognosis of small hepatocellular carcinoma (less than 3 cm) after percutaneous acetic acid injection: study of 91 cases. Hepatology 1996;23: 994–1002.
21. Ohnishi K, Yoshioka H, Kosaka K, Toshima K, Nishiyama J, Kameda C, Ito S, Fujiwara K. Treatment of hypervascular small hepatocellular carcinoma with ultrasound-guided percutaneous acetic acid injection: comparison with segmental transcatheter arterial embolization. Am J Gastroenterol 1996;91:2574–2579.

22. Child CG III. The liver and portal hypertension. Philadelphia, Pennsylvania: W.B. Saunders, 1964.
23. Kaplan EL, Meier P. Nonparametric estimation from incomplete observation. J Am Stat Assoc 1958;53:457–487.
24. Peto R, Pike MC, Armitage P, Breslow NE, Cox PR, Howard SV, Mantel N, Mcpherson K, Peto J, Smith PG. Design and analysis of randomized clinical trials requiring prolonged observation of each patient. II. Analysis and Examples. Br J Cancer 1977;35:1–39.
25. Okuda K, Musha H, Nakajima J, Kubo Y, Shimokawa Y, Nagasaki Y, Sawa Y, Jinnouchi S, Kaneko T, Obata H, Hisamitu T, Motoike Y, Okazaki N, Kojiro M, Sakamoto K. Clinicopathological features of hepatocellular carcinoma: a study of 26 cases. Cancer 1977;40:1240–1245.
26. Nakajima O. Pathological study on early hepatocellular carcinoma – A study of capsule and septum formation. Acta Hepatol Jpn 1989;30:28–34. (in Japanese)
27. Torimura T. Mechanism of the fibrous capsular formation surrounding hepatocellular carcinoma – immunohistochemical analysis. Acta Hepatol Jpn 1989;30:1596–1605 (In Japanese)
28. Utsunomiya T, Matsumata T, Adachi E, Honda H, Sugimachi K. Limitations of current preoperative liver imaging techniques for intrahepatic metastatic nodules of hepatocellular carcinoma. Hepatology 1992;16:694–701.
29. Rizzi P, Kane PA, Ryder SD et al. Accuracy of radiology in detection of hepatocellular carcinoma before liver transplantation. Gastroenterology 1994;107:1425–1429.
30. Takayama T, Makuuchi M, Hirohashi S, Sakamoto M, Okazaki N, Takayasu K, Kosuge T, Motoo Y, Yamzaki S, Hasegawa H. Malignant transformation of adenomatous hyperplasia to hepatocellular carcinoma. Lancet 1990;336:1150–1153.

Progress in Hepatology, Volume 3.
Hepatocellular Carcinoma.
M. Yamanaka, G. Toda and T. Tanaka, editors.

Development of percutaneous hot water injection therapy as the treatment of hepatocellular carcinoma

Takahiro Yamasaki[1], Akira Kato[1], Yuhki Yamaguchi[1], Fumie Kurokawa[1], Yoshiko Yabushita[2], Shuji Mizumachi[2] and Kiwamu Okita[1]
[1]First Department of Internal Medicine, Yamaguchi University, Yamaguchi, Japan; and [2]Department of Gastroenterology, Shimonoseki City Hospital, Yamaguchi, Japan

Abstract. We have examined percutaneous hot water injection therapy (PHoT) for hepatocellular carcinomas (HCCs). We conducted PHoT to nine cases of HCCs (18 nodules), in which we noticed complete necroses in 15 out of 17 nodules (88.2%) but did not recognize any serious complication. When we compared the PHoT group with the group undergoing percutaneous ethanol injection therapy (PEIT) of HCCs of <3 cm, we found that the number of therapies conducted could be reduced in the PHoT group, and no significant difference was observed in the therapeutic effect. In addition, in the PHoT group, the pain seemed to be lower.

When we conducted PHoT to tumor thrombi in the first branch of the portal vein of two cases, temporary improvements were observed. In addition, because the therapy was simple with less complication, PHoT to tumor thrombi could be considered as a part of effective multidisciplinary treatments. We conducted percutaneous hot water microwave coagulation therapy (PHMCT) in six cases of HCCs (six nodules) with <3 cm, in which we recognized no serious complication and found an enlarged necrosis area with the injection of 15 ml or more of hot water. A new development of PHoT treatment could be expected for HCC.

Keywords: hepatocellular carcinoma (HCC), percutaneous hot water microwave coagulation therapy (PHMCT), percutaneous hot water injection therapy (PHoT), tumor thrombus in the first branch of the portal vein, ultrasonography.

Introduction

The efficacy of percutaneous ethanol injection therapy (PEIT) to small hepatocellular carcinomas (HCCs) has already been reported [1]. However, the volume of hot water injected at one time is limited in PEIT, and there are cases in which the therapy has to be interrupted because of pain after injection. Recently, percutaneous hot water injection therapy (PHoT) was developed for small HCCs and reported effective because the number of times needed to conduct therapies and the side effects could be reduced [2]. In the present study, we have examined the treatment of HCCs by PHoT, and our findings will be reported in this paper.

Address for correspondence: Takahiro Yamasaki MD, First Department of Internal Medicine, Yamaguchi University, 1144 Kogusi, Ube, Yamaguchi 755, Japan. Tel.: +81-836-22-2241. Fax: +81-836-22-2240.

Patients and Methods

PHoT for HCCs

The subjects were of nine cases (18 nodules) of HCCs except for one case of HBsAg positive (case 8); all others were positive for HCV antibody (Table 1). The underlying liver disease was liver cirrhosis in eight patients and chronic hepatitis in one patient (case 1).

In conducting PHoT, we punctured the tumor percutaneously and transhepatically used an ultrasonically guided 21G needle (PEIT needle, Hakko Medical Products) and injected boiling hot physiological saline of 95°C. From the technical standpoint, we had immersed the glass syringe of 20 ml in boiling physiological saline, and filled the PEIT needle with hot water in advance so that the temperature would not be lowered. In one PHoT, we punctured a tumor 1–3 times. The volume of hot water injected was 25 ml maximum. After the treatment, the patient was kept at rest on the bed for 4 hours and the treatments were conducted twice a week. Informed consent was obtained from the patients before the procedure was performed.

The entire volume of hot water to inject was calculated by injecting 10 ml hot water into the HCC of 35 mm for case 1, in which we recognized the coagulation necrosis of 30% on the maximum split surface made by the surgery. Thus we set

Table 1. Characteristics of patients with HCC treated by PHoT.

Case No	Age/Sex	Site/Size (mm)	Clinical stage	Volume of hot water (ml)	Frequency of PHoT
1.	59/M	S7/35 × 33	I	10	1
2.	61/M	S7/37 × 35	I	59	4
		S6/10 × 7		24.5	3
		S8/17 × 9		12.5(+18.7)	1(+3)
		S7/12 × 10[a]		30	2
3.	74/F	S4/12 × 8	II	10	1
		S7/10 × 10		10	1
4.	72/F	S6/14 × 10	II	27(+35)	3(+4)
		S3/19 × 11[a]		21	3
		S2/16 × 14[a]		28	3
5.	64/M	S6/28 × 26	II	32	4
6.	54/M	S6/24 × 18	II	51.5(+15.5)	4(+2)
		S8/18 × 17		27(+26)	3(+3)
		S5/25 × 23[a]		78	4
7.	75/F	S4/44 × 43	II	200	10
		S5/25 × 22		49	4
8.	53/M	S7/30 × 24	III	72	5
9.	70/M	S5/13 × 11	II	31	2

[a]Recurrence nodule; ( ): additional treatment.

the volume at about 20 ml for the tumor having the diameter of 2 cm and about 60 ml for the tumor having the diameter of 3 cm.

To determine the therapeutic effect, we examined the lesion by the biopsy after the therapy as much as possible and the dynamic CT scans before and after the therapy. As a criterion for determining the therapeutic effect (TE), we used the standard of the Liver Cancer Study Group of Japan (Acta Hepatol Jpn 1994;35:193–205). In other words, we evaluated the TE according to the following five stages: TE V – necrotic effect of 100%; TE IV – necrotic effect of more than 50% and less than 100%; TE III – necrotic effect of more than 25% and less than 50%; TE II – necrotic effect of less than 25%; and TE I – regardless of the necrotic effect, the tumor increased by more than 25%.

We also examined the PHoT group (15 nodules) and the PEIT group (32 nodules) of HCCs of <3 cm we had experienced before on the number of times conducting the therapies, the entire volume injected, volume injected at one time, the pain as side effect and the therapeutic effects. PEIT was performed according to the method reported previously [1]. The total volume of ethanol injected in PEIT was determined according to the criteria proposed by Ebara et al. [1]. The total volume of ethanol injected was 15 to 20 ml in tumors with a diameter of 2 cm and 25 to 30 ml in tumors with a diameter of 3 cm. The volume of ethanol infused per injection ranged from 2 to 6 ml.

PHoT to the tumor thrombus in first branch of the portal vein of HCC

The subjects were two cases of HCCs complicated with tumor thrombi in the first branches of the portal vein (Vp3 [3]).

Case 1. Sixty-two years old male. On June 27, 1994, a massive type HCC was observed in the right lobe of liver accompanied by tumor thrombus in the trunk of the portal vein in the abdominal angiography. After three chemolipiodolizations, recanalization of the portal trunk and a shrunk intrahepatic tumor were observed. However, because the tumor thrombus in the right first branch of the portal vein did not show improvement, the patient was hospitalized on July 18, 1995 (clinical stage II [3]).

Case 2. Sixty-three years old male. On January 10, 1992, five nodules of HCC having the maximum diameter of 20 mm were observed in the anterior and posterior segments of liver in the abdominal angiography. After a chemolipiodolization, the tumor was found to have been disappeared. However from September 1993, recurrences of tumors in liver were observed and PHoT was conducted each time the tumor was found. As a tumor thrombus was observed in the left branch of the portal vein by the MRI conducted on December 8, 1995, the patient was hospitalized on December 18. (Clinical stage I [3]).

To conduct the PHoT, we punctured the tumor thrombus percutaneously and transhepatically using an ultrasonically guided PEIT needle, and we locally injected the boiling hot physiological saline. We began injecting from the peripheral side and gradually moved closer to the porta hepatis. In one PHoT, we punctured the tumor thrombus once and injected maximum of 20 ml. We conducted the treatment twice a week. Informed consent was obtained from the patients before the procedure was performed.

Percutaneous microwave coagulation therapy (PMCT) in combination with PHoT; percutaneous hot water microwave coagulation therapy (PHMCT) for HCCs

The subjects were six cases of HCCs with six nodules having the diameter <3 cm. Except for one case of HBsAg positive, other cases were HCV antibody positive. The underlying liver disease was liver cirrhosis in all patients.

When conducting percutaneous microwave coagulation therapy (PMCT), we used Microtase (HS-15M by Heiwa Denshi Kogyo) and the microwave electrode of 25 cm long and 1.6 mm thick.

As the therapeutic procedure, we used PHoT first, then conducted PMCT according to the method of Seki et al. [4]. The microwaves were applied for 60 s at 60 W, then dissociated for 20 s, and irradiated for 60 s at 60 W. After 1 week of PHMCT, we conducted a dynamic CT scan to examine the maximum necrosis area. Informed consent was obtained from patients before the procedure was performed.

Statistical analysis

The data was expressed by mean ± SD. The statistical analysis was examined using the t test, the χ^2 test, and the Mann-Whitney's U test. The accumulated survival rate was calculated by the Kaplan-Meier method [5]. The p value $\leqslant 0.05$ was considered significant.

Results

Table 1 shows the total volume of hot water injected and the number of times PHoT was conducted. The total volume of hot water injected was 10 to 200 ml, increasing with the diameter of the tumor. As for the number of times PHoT was conducted, the expected volume was reached at least 4 times for the tumor having the diameter <3 cm. However, in four out of 17 nodules (23.5%), because residual tumors were recognized after completion of the treatments except for case 1, additional PHoT was conducted.

As shown in Table 2, the therapeutic effects were recognized in 15 out of 17 nodules (88.2%) for TE V, one out of 17 nodules (5.9%) for TE IV, and one out of 17 nodules (5.9%) for TE I. Five out of eight cases survived, two cases (cases 5 and 7) died of cancer progression, and one case (case 8) died of hepatic dysfunction. The accumulated survival rate of eight cases were 72.9% for 1-year survival rate, and 58.3% for 3-year survival rate.

Table 2. Therapeutic effect of PHoT for treatment of HCC.

Case No.	Site/Size (mm)	Histological finding	Therapeutic effect (TE)	Prognosis (months)
1.	S7/35 × 33	moderate	–	Operation
2.	S7/37 × 35	moderate	V	42 alive
	S6/10 × 7	well	V	
	S8/17 × 9	well	V	
	S7/12 × 10[a]	moderate	V	
3.	S4/12 × 8	moderate	V	42 alive
	S7/10 × 10	well	V	
4.	S6/14 × 10	viable(+)	V	42 alive
	S3/19 × 11[a]	well	V	
	S2/16 × 14[a]	not done	V	
5.	S6/28 × 26	moderate	I	12 dead
6.	S6/24 × 18	moderate	V	38 alive
	S8/18 × 17	not done	V	
	S5/25 × 23[a]	moderate	V	
7.	S4/44 × 43	moderate	IV	25 dead
	S5/25 × 22	well	V	
8.	S7/30 × 24	moderate	V	2 dead
9.	S5/13 × 11	well	V	8 alive

[a]Recurrence nodule.

No serious complication was recognized. Fervescence of 38°C or less was found in 7.7% cases, and pain was observed in 21.7% cases, but both were transient. In two cases, increases of abdominal ascites were recognized, which were improved with the conservative treatment. In almost all cases, flares of skin were observed where punctures were made, but they did not require any treatment. Clear deterioration of hepatic function was not observed in any case.

Figure 1 shows case 6. We injected a total of 67 ml hot water with 6 times to the moderately differentiated HCC of 24 × 18 mm at S6. With the dynamic CT scan conducted at the completion of treatment, the tumor and the surrounding area were not enhanced. With the dynamic CT scan conducted at 3 months after treatment, the tumor had been shrunk.

We also compared the PHoT group with the PEIT group conducted to HCCs with the diameters <3 cm (Table 3). In the PHoT group, although they had unfavorable factors such as having a larger diameter of tumors and a larger number of moderately differentiated HCCs from histological differentiation, it was possible to reduce the number of PHoTs conducted because the increase of the volume of hot water to inject for one time was possible. There was no significant difference in the therapeutic effects. In the examination of the pain causing some problem as a kind of complication, the PHoT groups showed less pain while almost no significant difference was observed.

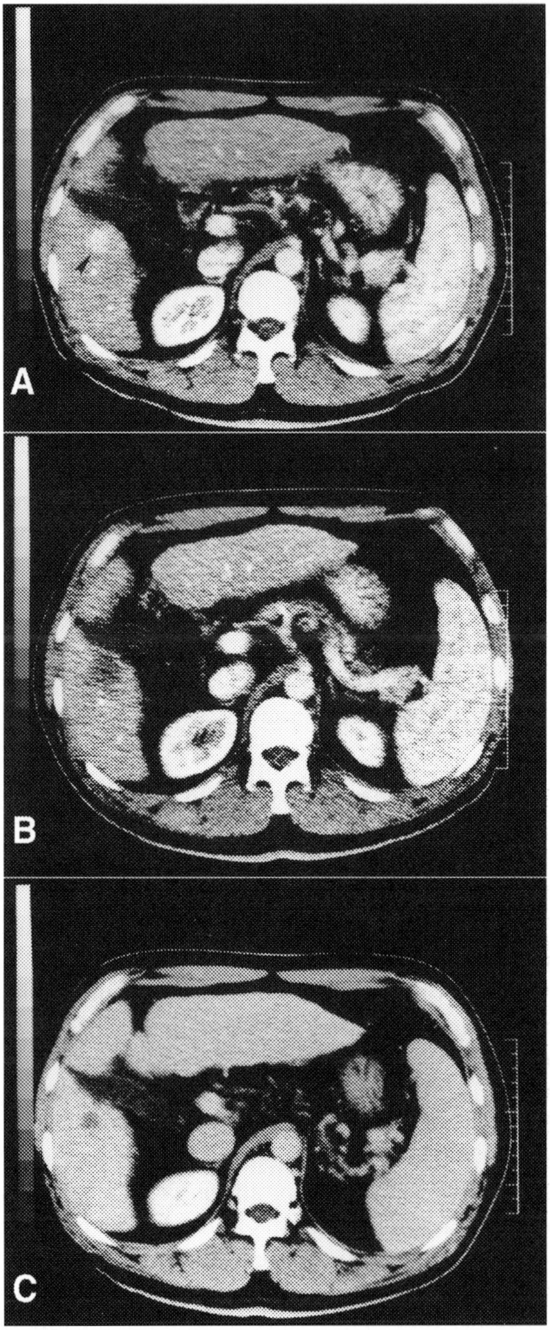

Fig. 1. Dynamic CT scans. **A**: Before treatment, the tumor site (arrow) is S6. **B**: The completion of treatment, the tumor and the surrounding area were not enhanced. **C**: Three months after treatment, the tumor had been shrunk.

Table 3. Comparison of PHoT group and PEIT group (HCC measuring less than 30 mm in diameter).

	PHoT (n = 15)	PEIT (n = 32)	p value
Tumor size (mm)	18 ± 6.8	14.6 ± 4.6	0.0380[a]
Histological finding			
well	6	29	0.0031[b]
moderate	6	2	
Frequency of therapy	3.7 ± 1.9	5.4 ± 1.4	0.0012[a]
Volume injected per therapy (ml)	10.9 ± 4.6	2.8 ± 0.9	0.0000065[a]
Total volume of hot water/ethanol (ml)	41.8 ± 23.2	15.3 ± 6.4	0.00057[a]
Side effect	14/55	65/174	0.0711[b]
severe pain(+)	(25.6%)	(37.4%)	
Therapeutic effect (TE)			
TE V	14 (93.3%)	31 (96.9%)	0.5791[c]
TE I	1 (6.7%)	1 (3.1%)	

[a]t test; [b]χ^2 test; [c]Mann-Whitney U test.

PHoT to the tumor thrombus of the first branch of the portal vein of HCC

Case 1. In the abdominal angiography before treatment, the first right branch of the portal vein was not observed. However, a large number of tumor stains with the maximum diameter of 30 mm were observed around the posterior segment, to which we conducted chemolipiodolization (40 mg of epirubicin, 8 mg of mitomycin C and 8 ml of lipiodol). An aspiration biopsy was conducted to the tumor thrombus. After confirming the malignant cells, we started PHoT to tumor thrombus in the first right branch of the portal vein after 2 weeks and injected a total of 75 ml hot water in six intervals . When we examined the power Doppler images (LOGIO500, GE, Yokogawa) before and after treatment, we observed a slight improvement of blood-flow in the first right branch of the portal vein (Fig. 2A,B). The patient in this case died of cancer progression at thirteen months after starting the treatment of tumor thrombus in the portal vein.

Case 2. In the abdominal angiography before treatment, the left branch of the portal vein was not observed. However, because a "thread and streaks" sign to the left branch of the portal vein was observed in the hepatic angiography, we conducted lipiodol-transcatheter arterial embolization (TAE) (20 mg of epirubicin, 4 mg of mitomycin C and 6 ml of lipiodol) (Fig. 3A). In the angiography conducted after lipiodol-TAE, the "thread and streaks" sign did not show any improvement.

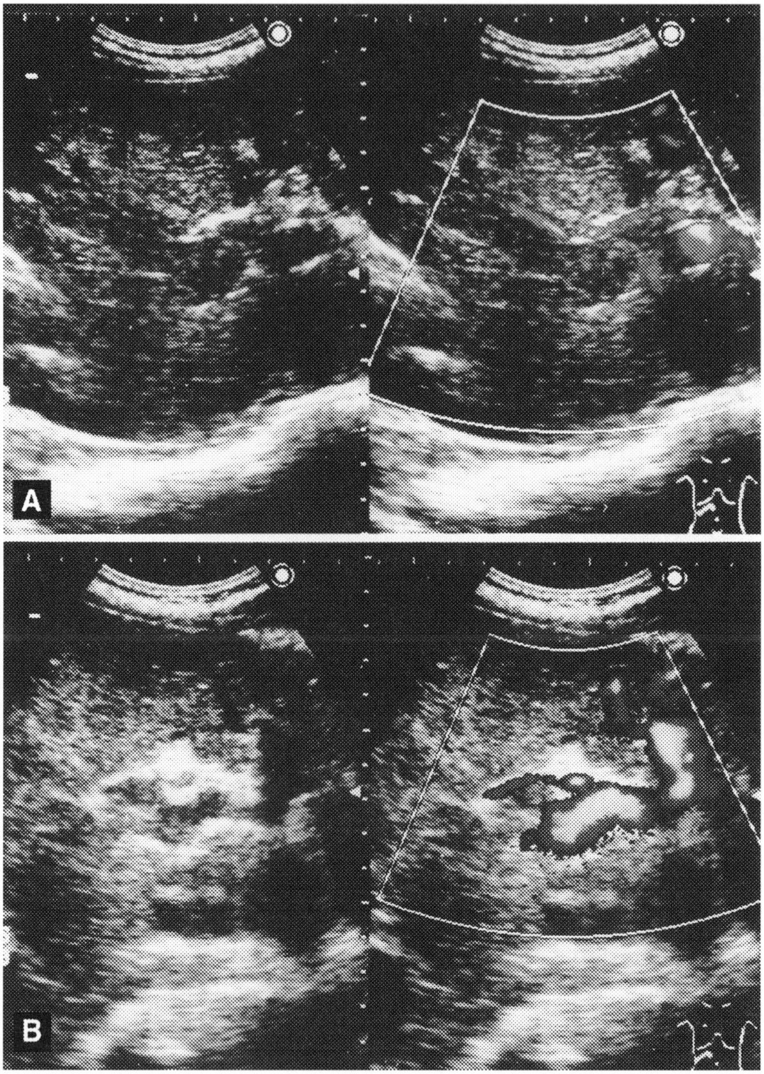

Fig. 2. Power Doppler images. **A**: Before treatment. **B**: After treatment, slight improvement of blood-flow in the first right branch of the portal vein was observed.

Thus, from 2 weeks afterwards, we started PHoT to the tumor thrombus in the left branch of the portal vein, and we injected a total of 126 ml hot water at 10 intervals. We also injected a total of 83.5 ml hot water at eight intervals to the HCC of 30 mm at S4. In the examination of power Doppler images before and after treatment, no improvement of blood-flow was observed in the left branch of the portal vein. However, at 2 months after starting the treatment (2 weeks after completion of PHoT to tumor thrombus), the left branch of the portal vein was not depicted in the abdominal angiography, and the "thread and streaks" sign disappeared

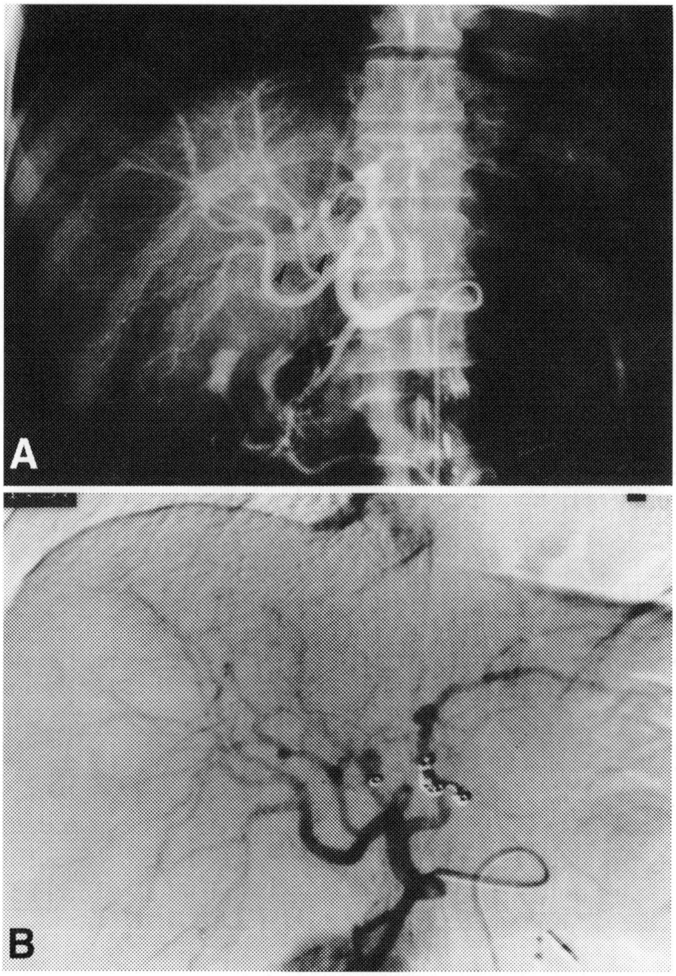

Fig. 3. The abdominal angiography. **A**: Before treatment, a thread and streaks sign (arrow) up to the left branch of the portal vein was observed in the hepatic angiography. **B**: At two months after starting the treatment, the thread and streaks sign disappeared in the hepatic angiography.

(Fig. 3B). The patient in this case has survived at present for 14 months after starting the treatment of tumor thrombus in the portal vein.

In the above-mentioned two cases, no severe side effect was observed and no fervescence or deterioration of hepatic function was observed except for the temporary pain and the ardor at the time of injection.

Percutaneous hot water microwave coagulation therapy (PHMCT) for HCCs (Table 4)

Except for case 5, we conducted PHMCT twice for each case. Enlarged necrosis

Table 4. Characteristics of patients HCC treated by PHMCT.

Case No.	Age/Sex	Site/Size (mm)	Histological finding	Clinical stage	Volume of hot water (ml)	Necrosis area (mm)
1.	62/M	S4/25 × 18	moderate	II	1st:7.5 2nd:5	20 × 20[a] 20 × 20[b]
2.	46/M	S8/20 × 16	well	I	1st:10 2nd:15	16 × 16[a] 20 × 16[b]
3.	69/F	S7/13 × 11	moderate	II	1st:10 2nd:10	30 × 16[a] 20 × 10[b]
4.	47/M	S6/18 × 16	well	III	1st:15 2nd:1.5	32 × 20[a] 36 × 20[b]
5.	63/M	S6/13 × 12	well	I	1st:20	28 × 16[a] 16 × 10[b]
6.	63/M	S7/20 × 19	well	II	1st:20 2nd:20	24 × 24[a] 24 × 18[b]

[a]1 week after PHMCT; [b]1 month after PHMCT.

areas were suggested with the increase of injected volume: cases 1 to 3, to which the volume of injected hot water was less than 10 ml, had the necrosis areas of 20 × 20, 16 × 16 and 30 × 16 mm, respectively; cases 4 to 6, to which the volume of injected hot water was more than 15 ml, had the necrosis areas of 32 × 20, 28 × 16 and 24 × 24 mm, respectively. Residual tumors were observed in cases 1 and 2, to which we conducted additional PHMCT.

As the complication, hemothrax was observed in one case (case 2), which improved conservatively, ardors were found in all cases, pains were found in 73% cases, and fervescences of less than 38°C were observed in 45% cases. In the transition of aspartate aminotransferase (AST) before and after treatment, increases of AST were observed in almost all cases, but no marked increase was observed.

Figure 4 shows the CT scan of single treatment with PMCT. To the well-differentiated HCC having the diameter of 8 mm at S7, we conducted PMCT for 120 seconds at 60 W, then took the dynamic CT at 1 week after treatment. The maximum necrosis area was 20 × 16 mm. On the other hand, with PHMCT, we conducted PHoT with 20 ml hot water and PMCT to the well-differentiated HCC of 20 × 19 mm at S7, then took the dynamic CT at 1 week after treatment. The maximum necrosis area was 24 × 24 mm (Fig. 5).

Discussion

With the recent advancement of image diagnosis and the development of PEIT, prognoses of HCCs have been drastically improved. However, recurrences of HCCs have been found at a high rate which need treatment each time the recurrence is found and repeated PEIT is possible. In other words, with the side effect of pain in PEIT, interruption of treatment has often been experienced. Recently,

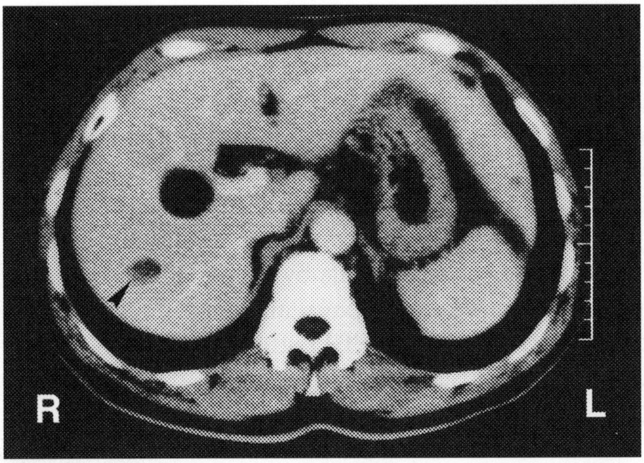

Fig. 4. Dynamic CT scan at one week after PMCT. The tumor (arrow) site is S7. PMCT was conducted for 120 s at 60 W. The maximum necrosis area was 20 × 16 mm.

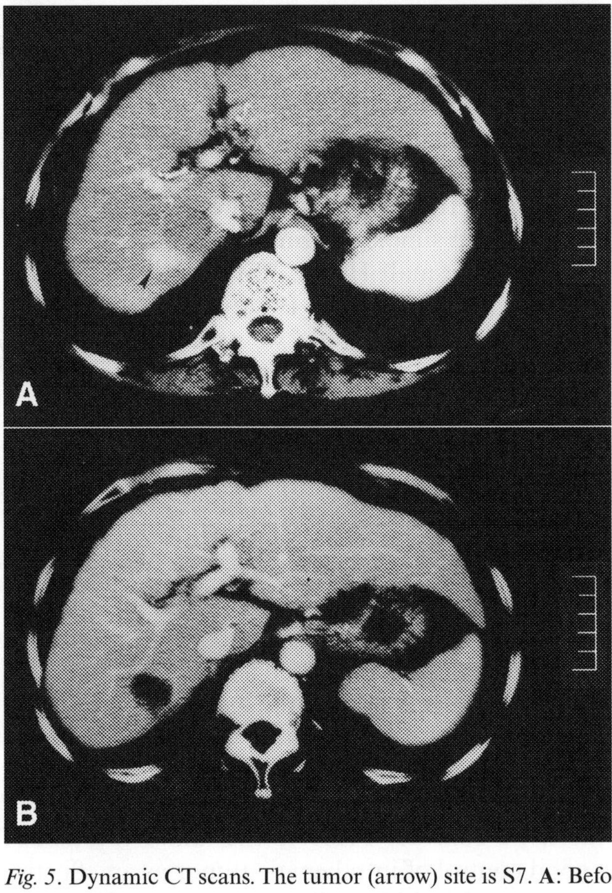

Fig. 5. Dynamic CT scans. The tumor (arrow) site is S7. **A**: Before treatment. **B**: One week after treatment. PHoT with 20 ml hot water and PMCT (PHMCT) was conducted. The maximum necrosis area was 24 × 24 mm.

PHoT to HCCs has been developed, in which the number of treatments conducted and the side effects have been reduced; this therapy was reported effective [2]. In comparing PHoT with PEIT, we reported that it was possible to reduce the number of times to conduct PHoT and the side effects [6]. In the present study, we added the cases and made examination to find that although the PHoT group had unfavorable factors such as having larger diameter of tumors and having larger number of moderately differentiated HCCs from histological differentiation, it was possible to reduce the number of treatments by increasing the volume of hot water to inject at one time. With regard to the pain, although no significant difference was observed between the PHoT and the PEIT groups, we found lesser pains in the PHoT group. In addition, because there was no significant difference on the therapeutic effect, the cases in which the continuation of PEIT was impossible due to the side effect can be considered as the first indication of PHoT. However, the period for observing the prognosis was still too short to draw a conclusion on the efficacy of PHoT, also there was an insufficient number of cases required for further examinations.

We are the first to report PHoT on tumor thrombus in the first branch of the portal vein of HCC (Vp3) [3]. The prognosis of HCC accompanied by Vp3 is poor, and many cases show resistance to the treatment. Recently, it was reported that repeated arterial infusion chemotherapy using a subcutaneously transplanted reservoir was conducted in the case of Vp3, in which the prognosis was improved [7]. However, the treatment was not directly conducted to the tumor thrombus in the portal vein. Thus, a direct and more simple treatment is expected. On the other hand, PEIT is direct and simple for small HCCs. PEIT conducted to the tumor thrombi in portal veins has been reported [8,9]. However, PEIT is not an established therapeutic method yet. In the present study, we paid attention to the advantages of PHoT in reducing the number of times required to conduct the therapy and avoid the side effects. We also conducted PHoT to the tumor emboli of portal veins in two cases. In case 1, although temporarily, an improved portal blood-flow was observed in the power Doppler images before and after PHoT; and in case 2, the disappearance of "thread and streaks" sign was observed before and after PHoT. Thus, we have come to consider that PHoT to the tumor thrombus in the portal vein is effective. As for the advantages of PHoT to the tumor thrombus in the portal vein, it is impossible to simply compare the number of treatments with the PEIT [8] because the entire volume to inject depends on the degree of tumor thrombus. However, the side effect is slight in the cases undergoing PHoT. Thus, the therapeutic effects almost the same as those could be obtained by PEIT. Because we used PHoT in combination with the therapeutic method by interventional radiology (IVR) to both two cases, we cannot report the single therapeutic effect of PHoT. However, because the hepatic function of these cases was relatively favorable, we consider PHoT to the tumor thrombi of portal veins of the cases having good control of intrahepatic tumor as an effective therapeutic method, that can be a part of multidisciplinary treatment due to the reduced side effects and simple treatments.

As the thermal coagulation occurs with the increase of the temperature of water molecules existing in tissues, it is possible to obtain a certain necrosis area by the microwave coagulation therapy (MCT). Recently, with the microwave electrode developed by Seki et al. (25 mm long and 1.6 mm thick), it has become possible to conduct the ultrasonically guided microwave irradiation. With the twice irradiations of 60 s at 60 W, necrosis area with the longer diameter of about 20 mm and the shorter diameter of 15 mm was reported [4]. In order to enlarge the necrosis area with one microwave irradiation, we designed PHMCT. In other words, with the combined use of the PHoT, we assumed two mechanisms, one of which is to have the coagulation necrosis effect by PHoT itself, and the other is to have the reinforced effect of PMCT by reinforcing the water molecules in tissues. With the injection volume of less than 10 ml in PHoT, the above-mentioned reinforced effect of necrosis was not frequently observed. Thus, an injection of 15 ml or more is considered necessary. Because what we have obtained is the preliminary data, we need more examinations. With regard to the side effects, there was not much difference seen by using only PMCT, and this method can be considered to be quite safe.

We could not determine whether PHoT was superior to PEIT, but if the advantages of reduced side effects and the number of times it takes to conduct the treatment are taken into consideration, PHoT can be said to be prospective in the future. Because our present data are still preliminary, we would like to be able to examine more cases.

References

1. Ebara M, Ohoto M, Sugiura N et al. Percutaneous ethanol injection for the treatment of small hepatocellular carcinoma. Study of 95 patients. J Gastroenterol Hepatol 1990;5:616–626.
2. Honda N, Guo Q, Uchida H et al. Percutaneous hot saline injection therapy for hepatic tumor: an alternative to percutaneous ethanol injection therapy. Radiology 1994;190:53–57.
3. Liver Cancer Study Group of Japan. The general rules for the clinical and pathological study of primary liver cancer. (in Japanese) 3rd edn. Tokyo: Kimbara, 1992;18–20.
4. Seki T, Wakabayashi M, Nakagawa T et al. Ultrasonically guided percutaneous microwave coagulation therapy for small hepatocellular carcinoma. Cancer 1994;74:817–825.
5. Kaplan EL, Meier P. Nonparametic estimation from incomplete observations. J Am Stat Assoc 1958;53:457–481.
6. Yamasaki T, Matsuzaki U, Irie K et al. Percutaneous hot water injection therapy (PHoT) for treatment of hepatocellular carcinoma: a comparison with percutaneous ethanol injection therapy (PEIT). Int Hepatol Commun 1995;3:305–309.
7. Minoyama A, Yoshikawa M, Ebara M et al. Study on repeated arterial infusion chemotherapy with a subcutaneously implanted reservoir for advanced hepatocellular carcinoma. J Gastroenterol 1995;30:356–366.
8. Yamasaki T, Nishikawa J, Irie K et al. A case of hepatocellular carcinoma (HCC) with long term survival by transcatheter arterial embolization (TAE) and percutaneous ethanol injection therapy (PEIT) to tumor thrombus in the right portal vein (Vp3). Acta Hepatol Jpn 1994;35: 448–454.
9. Livraghi T, Grigioni W, Mazziotti A et al. Percutaneous alcohol injection of portal thrombosis in hepatocellular carcinoma: a new possible treatment. Tumori 1990;76:394–397.

Progress in Hepatology, Volume 3.
Hepatocellular Carcinoma.
M. Yamanaka, G. Toda and T. Tanaka, editors.

Outcome of transcatheter arterial embolization for hepatocellular carcinoma

Mariko Itsubo
Department of Internal Medicine (1), Jikei University School of Medicine, Tokyo, Japan

Abstract. Transcatheter arterial embolization (TAE) has been playing an important part in the treatment for hepatocellular carcinoma (HCC). In most of our cases, it has been performed as lipiodol chemoembolization; the mixture of lipiodol and an antitumor agent (chiefly, epidoxorubicin) and small particles of gelatin sponge. The 1- and 3-year cumulative survival rates of the patients with solitary tumor < 5.0 cm in diameter treated between 1991 and 1996 were 93.1 and 73.3%, respectively. The 5-year survival rate may be estimated at approximately 50%. Segmental or subsegmental TAE brought the broad application to the patients with various backgrounds. It was effectively applicable to small-sized HCC less than 2.0 cm in diameter when tumor showed hypervascularity. The 5-year cumulative survival rate was 50.9%. Also, it was effectively and safely applicable to the patients with tumor thrombosis in the main track of the portal vein when efficient intrahepatic portal blood flow was anticipated. Recently, a lipophilic antitumor agent has been available for arterial infusion of HCC in order to retain with lipiodol in the tumor for a long time. As a result of our preliminary study, further clinical study will be needed to elucidate the significance of this agent.

Keywords: epidoxorubicin, lipiodol chemoembolization, portal vein invasion, small-sized HCC, SMANCS, super selective TAE, transcatheter arterial embolization, transcatheter arterial infusion chemotherapy, zinostatin stymalamer.

Introduction

Transcatheter arterial embolization (TAE) for hepatocellular carcinoma (HCC) [1] has been widely performed in unresectable cases, and it is an important procedure in the multidisciplinary treatment. In general, the conception of TAE includes chemoembolization and lipiodol chemoembolization. Although complete necrosis of the whole tumor is sometimes obtained by TAE alone, tumor extension including intra- or extracapsule invasion and portal vein involvement will be hardly affected by embolization [2,3].

Many patients with unresectable HCC have been treated by TAE in our department since 1983. It was not easy to insert the conventional pre-shaped catheters including RH, RC2 and Mikaelsson into the further distal branches of the right or left hepatic artery in the first several years, therefore it was almost impossible to accomplish the segmental or subsegmental TAE without damaging nontumor area. The recent advancement of catheter and guidewire has allowed a coaxial

Address for correspondence: Mariko Itsubo, Department of Internal Medicine (1), Jikei University School of Medicine, 3-25-8, Nishishinbashi, Minato-ku, Tokyo 105, Japan. Tel.: +81-3-3433-1111. Fax: +81-3-3435-1922.

approach through the conventional catheters, and a tip of the fine catheter can reach smaller feeding arteries. In fact, it has resulted in the improvement in the outcome of TAE.

In this paper, the outcome of TAE is reviewed mainly for the patients in some conditions, including those with small-size tumor, with portal vein invasion, and using a lipophilic antitumor agent, experienced in our department.

Present state of the outcome of TAE for HCC

The applicable patients and materials of TAE in our department are shown in Table 1. Almost all the patients coexist with liver cirrhosis. The patients were evaluated for their hepatic functional reserve in the clinical stage, the criteria designed by the Liver Cancer Study Group of Japan [4]. The patients in stage I or II can be applicants for TAE, in principle. TAE, as a well-known fact, is not applicable to the patient with the portal trunk obstruction without efficient intrahepatic portal blood flow. TAE has been performed as lipiodol chemoembolization in most of our cases; first, the mixture of lipiodol and an antitumor agent (chiefly, 40–60 mg epidoxorubicin) was infused via the catheter into targeted arterial branches, then the vessels were completely occluded by small particles of gelatin sponge. These procedures were performed in the region of segment or subsegment of the liver, corresponding to the tumor growth (Fig. 1).

The outcome was not sufficient in the early years, although it was superior to the outcome of arterial chemolipiodolization (infusion of the mixture of lipiodol and an antitumor agent, alone), and the 5-year survival rate was less than 10% [5]. Lately, the outcome of TAE has been improving probably owing to diagnosis in the early stage and super selective catheterization for treatment. Figure 2 shows the cumulative survival curves of the patients in our department initially treated by TAE between April 1991 and March 1996 as analyzed by the

Table 1. Transcatheter arterial embolization for hepatocellular carcinoma.

Patients: Clinical stage[a] I or II, in principle
 Ascites; none or controllable
 Serum total bilirubin <3.0 mg/dl
 Serum albumin $\geqslant 3.0$ g/dl
 ICG R15 $\leqslant 40\%$
 Prothrombin time $\geqslant 50\%$
  At least 4 items must be satisfied
 Not coexisted with portal trunk obstruction
Materials: Antitumor agent (epidoxorubicin, mitomycin C or SMANCS)
 + Lipiodol
 + Small particles of gelatin sponge

[a]There are three clinical stages of the host of liver cancer classified according to the clinical and laboratory findings in "the general rules for the clinical and pathological study of primary liver cancer" by the Liver Cancer Study Group of Japan [4]. Clinical stage I or II means the hepatic functional reserve is relatively good in the patient.

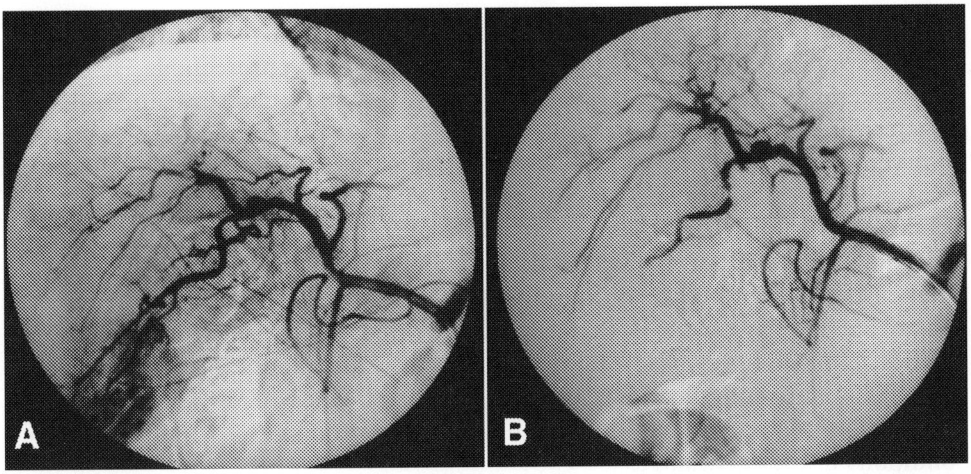

Fig. 1. Subsegmental TAE for HCC in the segment 6. **A**: Pretreatment hepatic arteriogram. **B**: Hepatic arteriogram after TAE. Posteroinferior branch was completely occluded.

Kaplan-Meier method. The 1- and 3-year cumulative survival rates of all patients were 82.7 and 38.2%, respectively. The 5-year survival rate may be estimated at approximately 20%. The 1- and 3-year survival rates of the patients with solitary tumor < 5.0 cm in diameter were 93.1 and 73.3%, respectively. The 5-year survival rate may be estimated at approximately 50%. These results were not worse than those in other reports [6,7]. So far, many reports on the outcome of TAE

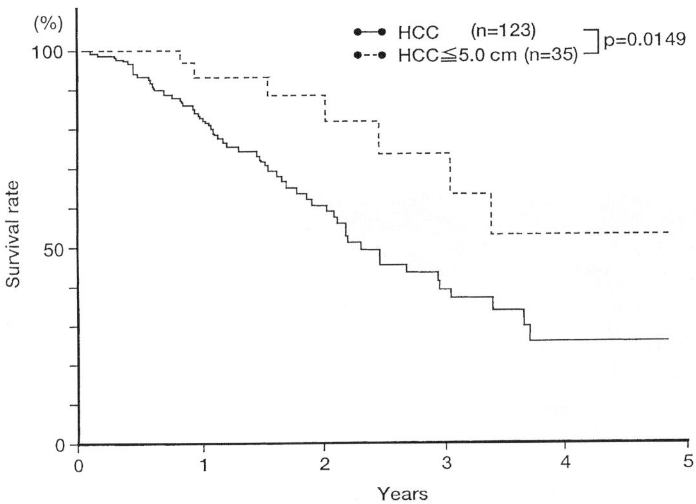

Fig. 2. Cumulative survival curves of HCC treated by TAE between April 1991 and March 1996. The 1- and 3-year survival rates of all patients were 82.7 and 38.2%, respectively. The 1- and 3-year survival rates of the patients with solitary tumor < 5.0 cm in diameter were 93.1 and 73.3%, respectively.

for HCC have been published in Japan, but some recent reports from Western countries support that TAE is an effective treatment for unresectable HCC [8,9].

Considerably, tumors became efficient necrosis in many cases by super selective catheterization, but on the other hand a few cases with rare complications were observed. One case suffered from hepatic biloma caused by injury of the intrahepatic bile duct due to occlusion of the peribiliary plexus in the anterosuperior artery (Fig. 3); another case suffered from subcutaneous necrosis in the upper abdominal wall caused by occlusion of the hepatic falciform artery [10]. In the latter case, the only mixture of lipiodol and the antitumor agent was used without gelatin sponge particles. Both cases were cured by conservative treatments. Besides nonspecific symptoms including nausea and abdominal pain, various side effects and complications after TAE are well known. We should carefully observe the treated patients during and after the procedure to find the morbid conditions in the early stage.

Outcome of TAE for solitary HCC <2.0 cm in diameter

The solitary HCC <5.0 cm in diameter may be the most efficient applicant of TAE [6,11]. Although small-size HCC <2.0 cm in diameter may be effectively treated by percutaneous ethanol injection therapy (PEIT) [12] in many unresectable cases, it would also obtain satisfactory therapeutic effect by TAE when the tumor shows enough arterial vascularity. Actually, the author reported that the 5-year cumulative survival rate was 50.9% as the outcome of TAE for the patients with small-size <2.0 cm in diameter hypervascular HCC treated between September 1983 and December 1994 [13]. The 1-, 3- and 5-year survival rates were 95.0, 59.4 and 50.9%, respectively. The survival curve was relatively superior to that of the patients with a tumor of 2.1 to 5.0 cm in diameter during the same observation period without statistical difference (Fig. 4). In that clinical study, the complete response rate including responders after repeated treatments was 20%, and it was almost equal to that of another group (patients with 2.1–5.0

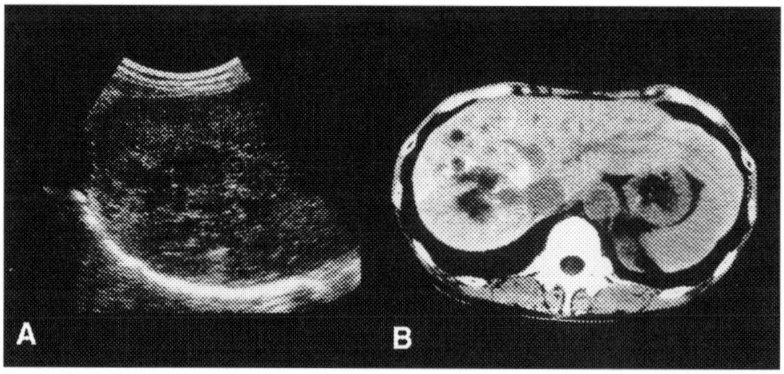

Fig. 3. **A**: Ultrasonography showed irregular hypoechoic lesion in the right hepatic lobe. **B**: CT showed an inhomogeneous density area caused by lipiodol accumulation and bile lake corresponding to the lesion by ultrasonography.

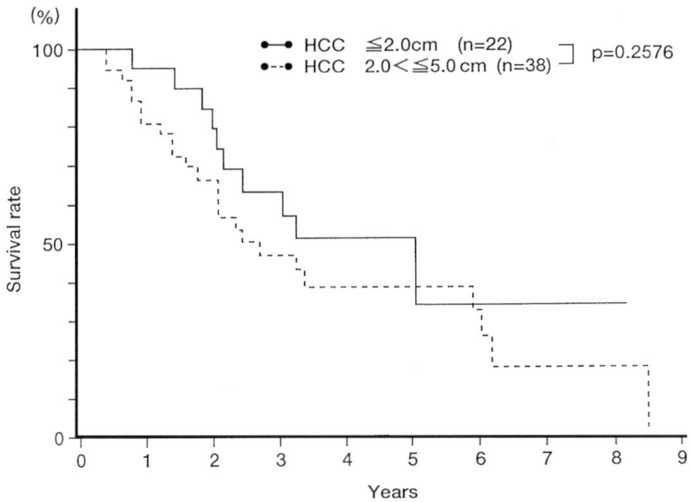

Fig. 4. Cumulative survival curves of solitary HCC < 5.0 cm in diameter treated by TAE between September 1983 and December 1994. The 1-, 3- and 5-year survival rates of small-size HCC < 2.0 cm in diameter were 95.0, 59.4 and 50.9%, respectively. The 1-, 3- and 5-year survival rates of HCC > 2.0 cm in diameter were 83.5, 50.9 and 41.5%, respectively.

cm in tumor size). Although the effect of TAE might be inferior to the effect of PEIT regarding the local control of small-size HCC, the survival rate was almost equal to the survival of the patients treated by PEIT; 49% at 5-year [14].

According to our experience [13], it seems that TAE with super selective catheterization is the effective treatment without severe side effects and complications even for solitary small-size HCC < 2.0 cm in diameter when tumor is detected as hypervascular lesion in the case without severe liver dysfunction. Even if complete tumor necrosis could not be observed after the initial TAE, repeated TAE was capable of leading complete necrosis in some cases. Similar evidence was given by another report [15]. Regarding the side effect, an increase in serum ALT activity or bilirubin was temporarily seen in approximately one-third of the cases. The incidence was relatively lower than that in another group (2.1—5.0 cm in tumor size).

TAE in the case of HCC with portal vein invasion

It is well known that the application of TAE for the patients with tumor thrombosis in the first branch or trunk of the portal vein is prohibited to prevent fatal hepatic failure caused by the treatment. However, if efficient intrahepatic portal blood flow is anticipated, TAE still has hope for such patients.

As the result of our retrospective study (Jan. 1990 — Dec. 1995) of the patients with tumor invasion in the main portal track stated above for comparing the survival curves of some therapeutic measures, including TAE, transcatheter arterial

Table 2. Treatment for patients with tumor invasion in the first branch or trunk of the portal vein.

	Supportive treatment (n = 15)	TAI (one shot) (n = 10)	TAI (reservoir) (n = 5)	TAE (n = 5)
Age (yr)	64.7 ± 10.3	59.6 ± 8.8	59.4 ± 11.4	59.6 ± 8.8
CS I/II/III	1/5/9	0/7/3	1/3/1	3/2/0
Tumor growth uni-/bilateral	6/9	3/7	4/1	2/3
Survival rate				
3 months	6.7%	40%	100%	100%
6 months	0	10%	20%	60%
1 year	0	0	0	40%

TAI = transcatheter arterial infusion chemotherapy; Age, values are mean ± SD; CS = clinical stage.

infusion chemotherapy (TAI, one shot), transcatheter arterial infusion chemotherapy using an implantable port (TAI, reservoir), or supportive therapy alone, it showed that the survival rate of TAE was superior to those of other therapeutic groups (Table 2). The backgrounds of the patients were not equal among these groups, therefore it was difficult to draw a conclusion. At least, 40% in 1-year survival rate was shown in only the group treated by TAE, although the survival of more than 1 year in most of the patients was not observed. There are few papers concerning the outcome of TAE for HCC with portal vein invasion, but recently, prolonged survival in HCC patients with peripheral (1st, 2nd or 3rd order branch) portal vein thrombosis has been seen [16].

Among these patients treated by TAE, one was operated successfully and no recurrence has been found during the 15 months after the operation. Figure 5

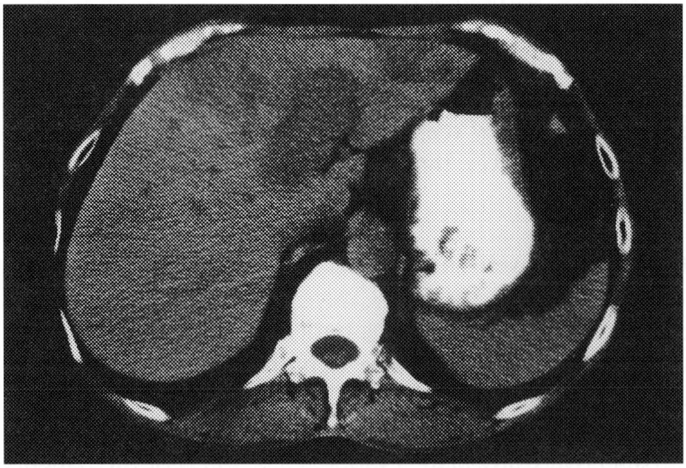

Fig. 5. CT showed two low-density lesions in the medial and lateral segments of the left hepatic lobe and remarkable portal tumor thrombosis in the porta hepatis.

shows the pretreatment picture of computed tomography of this patient. Tumors were located in the medial and lateral segments of the left lobe of the liver, and tumor thrombosis was found in the main portal track. The arterial portogram showed complete obstruction of the left branch and incomplete obstruction of the right branch and trunk of the portal vein. The hepatic arteriogram showed the "thread and streaks" sign [17] in the porta hepatis and arterio-portal communication with the right branch of the portal vein (Fig. 6). After 3 times of TAE during 6 months, the regression of the portal thrombosis and a decrease of serum alpha-fetoprotein level (26,000 to 700 ng/ml) were observed (Fig. 7). The patient underwent left-side hepatic lobectomy 8 months after the initial TAE.

Super selective TAE as subsegmental TAE may effectively and safely be applied to the patients with portal vein invasion, when intrahepatic portal blood flow and hepatic functional reserve are fully kept. Owing to the growth of portal vein invasion, an increase of degree of esophageal varices is observed [18,19]. Quite a few patients with advanced portal thrombosis die from rupture of the esophageal varices. Therefore, the risk of rupture from the esophageal varices may be reduced by suppression of the growth of portal thrombosis when effective TAE is performed, also it will contribute to the prolonged survival.

Outcome of TAE with a lipophilic antitumor agent

Antitumor agents used in TAE have been selected among hydrophilic compounds including doxorubicin, epidoxorubicin, mitomycin C and cisplatinum. Although lipiodol chemoembolization has been widely performed, these hydrophilic com-

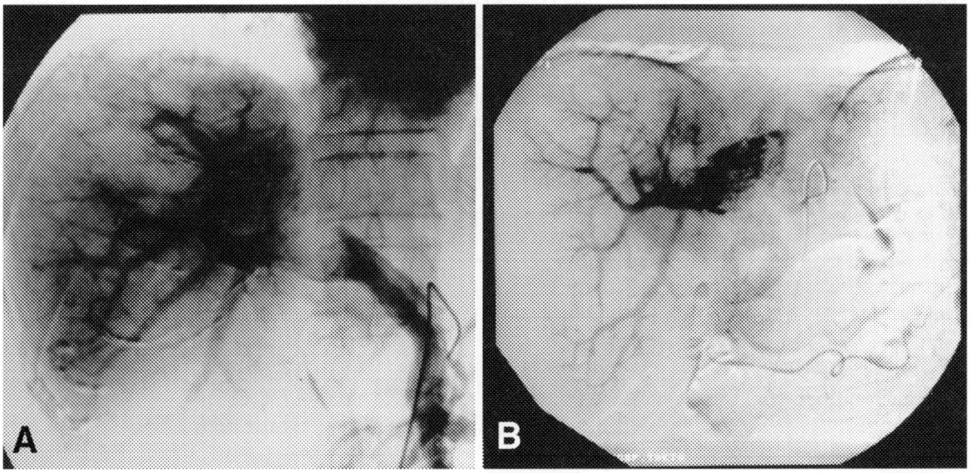

Fig. 6. **A**: Arterial portogram showed complete obstruction of the left branch of the portal vein and incomplete obstruction of the right branch and trunk of the portal vein. **B**: Left hepatic arteriogram showed the thread and streaks sign in the porta hepatis and arterioportal communication with the right branch of the portal vein.

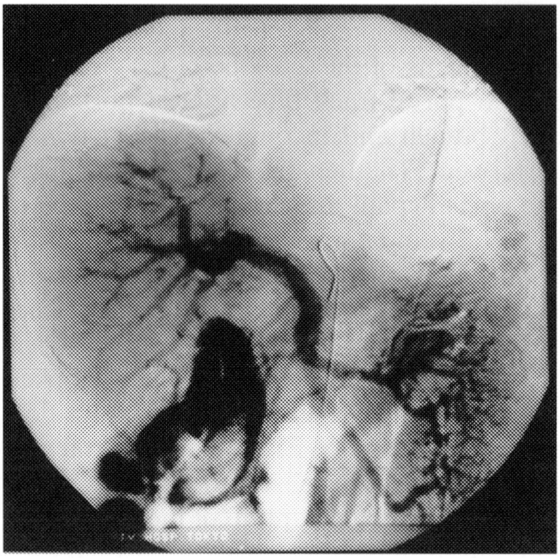

Fig. 7. Arterial portogram after 2 times of TAE showed regression of the tumor thrombosis in the right branch and trunk of the portal vein.

pounds may not essentially be suitable for retaining with lipiodol in the tumor for a long time. Recently, a lipophilic antitumor agent, zinostatin stymalamer (SMANCS) [20] has been available and are now widely used for arterial infusion for HCC.

The result of our comparative study of antitumor effect between the patients treated by initial TAE with SMANCS and the patients treated by TAE with epidoxorubicin showed no remarkable difference. In this study, 40 patients initially treated by TAE between January 1994 and December 1995 were evaluated (Table 3). Antitumor effect was assessed as a therapeutic effect by the criteria designed by the Liver Cancer Study Group of Japan [21]; it is classified into five grades

Table 3. Backgrounds of the patients.

	SMANCS (n = 15)	Epidoxorubicin (n = 25)
Age (yr)	60.9 ± 7.5	60.6 ± 10.9
Clinical stage I+II/III	13/2(87%)	22/3(88%)
Tumor growth		
T1+T2 / T3+T4[a]	10/5(67%)	17/8(68%)
single/multiple	9/6(60%)	17/8(68%)
Agent (mg)	3.5 ± 0.7	34.0 ± 16.6
LPD (ml)	5.4 ± 3.5	7.1 ± 5.1

[a]T factor in "the general rules for the clinical and pathological study of primary liver cancer" by the Liver Cancer Study Group of Japan [4]. T1+T2 means, briefly, a single tumor or multiple tumors with a maximum tumor diameter of 2 cm or less confined to one lobe without vascular invasion; T3+T4 means tumor growth is more progressive. LPD = lipiodol.

Table 4. Therapeutic effects (TEs)[a] after initial TAE.

	SMANCS (n = 15)	Epidoxorubicin (n = 25)
TE V	4	10
TE IV	8	12
TE III	1	0
TE II	2	3
TE I	0	0
TE V	4 (27%)	10(40%)
TE V+IV	12 (80%)	22(88%)

[a]The criteria designed by the Liver Cancer Study Group of Japan [21].
TE V = complete tumor necrosis or tumor regression.
TE IV = 50% $\leqslant$ tumor necrosis or regression $<100\%$.
TE III = 25% $\leqslant$ tumor necrosis or regression $<50\%$.
TE II = tumor necrosis or regression $<25\%$.
TE I = over 25% of tumor growth regardless of the degree of tumor necrosis.

evaluated by the imaging diagnosis. Mean dosages of SMANCS and epidoxorubicin were 3.5 and 34.0 mg, respectively. There was no significant difference of patients backgrounds including the tumor growth between the two groups. Over 50% of tumor necrosis was obtained in 80% (complete necrosis in 27%) of cases treated with SMANCS and in 88% (complete necrosis in 40%) of cases treated with epidoxorubicin (Table 4). Regarding the side effects, hematologic and hepatic toxicities were temporarily observed in approximately 60% and 70—80% respectively in both groups. There was no significant difference between the two groups (Table 5).

It is well known that HCC is one of the malignant neoplasms with poor response to the treatment with antitumor agents. The membrane protein, P-glycoprotein [22], plays an important role in multidrug resistance to cancer chemotherapy. Actually, many cases of untreated HCC show P-glycoprotein expression in tumor tissues [23]. Although the most effective factor for tumor necrosis by TAE including lipiodol chemoembolization seemed to be ischemic change by occlusion of feeding arteries, the effect of antitumor agent is expected to form a part of it. Therefore, antitumor agents should be carefully selected to improve the outcome of treatment. SMANCS was expected to improve therapeutic effect

Table 5. Hematologic and hepatic toxicities.

	SMANCS (n = 14)	Epidoxorubicin (n = 24)
Hematologic toxicity	8 (57%)	14 (58%)
Hepatic toxicity	10 (71%)	20 (83%)

Hematologic toxicity: over 25% of decrease in the number of WBC, RBC or thrombocyte compared with pretreatment level; Hepatic toxicity: over 50% of increase in the level of total bilirubin or ALT compared with pretreatment level.

by arterial infusion of the mixture with lipiodol for HCC [24]. This compound is not transported by P-glycoprotein. Although the results of our clinical study in the patients treated by arterial infusion of the mixture of lipiodol and antitumor agent is preliminary, antitumor effect by SMANCS was almost similar to that by epidoxorubicin (data not shown). It seems that additional arterial embolization using gelatin sponge particles may be needed to obtain more efficient antitumor effect even if this compound is used.

TAE, playing an important part of multidisciplinary treatment for HCC

Multidisciplinary performance is not an exception in treatment for HCC, and TAE is usually selected as the initial treatment for hypervascular unresectable tumors. In fact, it is expected to obtain considerable tumor necrosis by TAE. However, it is common knowledge that it is not easy to achieve the complete necrosis of the tumor by TAE alone. Therefore various additional therapeutic procedures have been performed including hyperthermia [25]. When tumor size is not so large, additional PEIT will be effective [26]. Although another treatment including hepatic resection was selected for the initial treatment, TAE has been widely performed for recurrence or regrowth tumors in many cases. Thus, various treatments are added in one patient during the course of the disease, therefore it is sometimes difficult to evaluate the efficacy of individual procedure. A recent paper [27] reported that the 5-year survival rate of the patients with HCC who received multidisciplinary treatment was 18%. The reason why the survival curve of the patients in the latter period of their study was better than that in the former period is probably due to improved techniques, including TAE. To achieve a better outcome of HCC, TAE should be carefully performed to prevent artificial vascular injury and excessive hepatic injury by delicate catheterization and selective embolization.

References

1. Yamada R, Sato M, Kawabata M, Nakatsuka H, Nakamura K, Takashima S. Hepatic artery embolization in 120 patients with unresectable hepatoma. Radiology 1983;148:397–401.
2. Sakurai M, Okamura J, Kuroda C. Transcatheter chemo-embolization effective for treating hepatocellular carcinoma: a histopathologic study. Cancer 1984;54:387–392.
3. Hsu HC, Wei TC, Tsang YM, Wu MZ, Lin YH, Chuang SM. Histopathologic assessment of resected hepatocellular carcinoma after transcatheter hepatic arterial embolization. Cancer 1986;57:1184–1191.
4. Liver Cancer Study Group of Japan. The general rules for clinical and pathological study of primary liver cancer. Jpn J Surg 1989;19:98–129.
5. Itsubo M, Hara M, Sakaguchi M, Kawabe T, Negishi M, Miyazaki H, Aoyama N, Asukata I, Kameda H. Prognosis and prognostic factors in the patients with unresectable hepatocellular carcinoma treated with transcatheter therapy. Tokyo Jikeikai Med J 1990;105:845–850. (in Japanese.)
6. Nishimura Y, Uchida H, Qiyong Guo, Matsuo N, Ohue S, Nishimine K, Sakaguchi H, Ohishi H, Yoshioka T, Fukui H, Tsujii T. Transcatheter arterial embolization (TAE) for 1,075 cases of hepatocellular carcinoma: evaluation of TAE using lipiodol mixed with anticancer agents focusing

on cumulative survival rate and 69 cases achieving 3-year survival. J Jpn Soc Cancer Ther 1992;26:2279–2289. (in Japanese.)

7. Taniguchi K, Nakata K, Kato Y, Sato Y, Hamasaki K, Tsuruta S, Nagataki S. Treatment of hepatocellular carcinoma with transcatheter arterial embolization: analysis of prognostic factors. Cancer 1994;73:1341–1345.
8. Bismuth H, Morino M, Sherlock D, Castaing D, Miglietta C, Cauquil P, Roche A. Primary treatment of hepatocellular carcinoma by arterial chemoembolization. Am J Surg 1992;163: 387–394.
9. Bronowicki JP, Vetter D, Dumas F, Boudjema K, Bader R, Weiss AM, Wenger JJ, Boissel P, Bigard MA, Doffoel M. Transcatheter oily chemoembolization for hepatocellular carcinoma: a 4-year study of 127 French patients. Cancer 1994;74:16–24.
10. Koike K, Itsubo M, Hara M, Enomoto Y, Okuda J, Hokari A, Okuaki Y, Sakaguchi M, Kawabe T, Toda G. A case of hepatocellular carcinoma with subcutaneous necrosis on upper abdominal wall after chemolipiodolization therapy. Acta Hepatol Jpn 1996;37:36–41. (in Japanese.)
11. Shimamura Y, Gunven P, Takenaka Y, Shimizu H, Shima Y, Akimoto H, Arima K, Takahashi A, Kitaya T, Matsuyama T, Hasegawa H. Combined peripheral and central chemoembolization of liver tumors: experience with lipiodol-doxorubicin and gelatin sponge (L-TAE). Cancer 1988; 61:238–242.
12. Ebara M, Ohto M, Sugiura N, Kita K, Yoshikawa M, Okuda K, Kondo F, Kondo Y. Percutaneous ethanol injection for the treatment of small hepatocellular carcinoma: study of 95 patients. J Gastroenterol Hepatol 1990;5:616–626.
13. Itsubo M, Sakaguchi M, Shimada N, Koike K, Okuda J, Enomoto Y, Tsuno S, Hokari A, Kawabe T, Negishi M, Toda G. Therapeutic effects of transcatheter arterial embolization using lipiodol mixed with antitumor agents for small hepatocellular carcinoma. J Jpn Soc Cancer Ther 1996;31:349–355. (in Japanese.)
14. Ebara M, Sugiura N, Yoshikawa M, Fukuda M, Sanada M, Ohto M. Nonsurgical treatment for hepatocellular carcinoma: indications and results. Kan-Tan-Sui 1994;29:341–348. (in Japanese.)
15. Ikeda K, Kumada H, Saitoh S, Arase Y, Chayama K. Effect of repeated transcatheter arterial embolization on the survival time in patients with hepatocellular carcinoma: an analysis by the Cox proportional hazard model. Cancer 1991;68:2150–2154.
16. Yen FS, Wu JC, Kuo BIT, Chiang JH, Chen TZ, Lee SD. Transcatheter arterial embolization for hepatocellular carcinoma with portal vein thrombosis. J Gastroenterol Hepatol 1995;10:237–240.
17. Okuda K, Musha M, Yoshida T, Kanda Y, Yamazaki T, Jinnouchi S, Moriyama Y, Kawaguchi S, Kubo Y, Shimokawa Y, Kojiro M, Kuratomi S, Nakashima T. Demonstration of growing casts of hepatocellular carcinoma in the portal vein by celiac angiography: the thread and streaks sign. Radiology 1975;117:303–309.
18. Nagasue N, Inokuchi K, Kobayashi M, Saku M. Hepatoportal arteriovenous fistula in primary carcinoma of the liver. Surg Gynecol Obstet 1977;145:504–508.
19. Murashima N, Arase Y, Ikeda K, Chayama K, Saitoh S, Suzuki Y, Tsubota A, Koide I, Kobayashi M, Kumada H. Endoscopic regression and evaluation of injection sclerotherapy for esophageal varices in case of hepatocellular carcinoma with portal vein invasion. Gastroenterol Endoscopy 1996;38:2379–2385. (in Japanese.)
20. Maeda H, Takeshita J, Kanamaru R. A lipophilic derivative of neocarzinostatin: a polymer conjugation of antitumor protein antibiotic. Int J Peptide Protein Res 1979;14:81–87.
21. Liver Cancer Study Group of Japan. Criteria of tumor response after nonsurgical treatment for liver cancer. Acta Hepatol Jpn 1994;35:193–205. (in Japanese.)
22. Juliano RL, Ling V. A surface glycoprotein in modulating drug permeability in Chinese hamster ovary cell mutants. Biochim Biophys Acta 1976;455:152–162.
23. Itsubo M, Ishikawa T, Toda G, Tanaka M. Immunohistochemical study of expression and cellular localization of the multidrug resistance gene product P-glycoprotein in primary liver carcinoma. Cancer 1994;73:298–303.

24. Konnno T, Maeda H, Iwai K. Tashiro S, Maki S, Morinaga T, Mochinaga M, Hiraoka T, Yokoyama I. Effect of arterial administration of high-molecular-weight anticancer agent SMANCS with lipid lymphographic agent on hepatoma: a preliminary report. Eur J Cancer Clin Oncol 1983;19:1053–1065.
25. Nagata Y, Abe M, Hiraoka M, Masunaga S, Akuta K, Nishimura Y, Takahashi M, Jo S, Koishi M. Radiofrequency hyperthermia and radiotherapy for hepatocellular carcinoma. In: Tobe T, Kameda H, Okudaira M, Ohto M, Endo Y, Mito M, Okamoto E, Tanikawa K, Kojiro M (eds) Primary Liver Cancer in Japan. Tokyo: Springer-Verlag, 1992;315–325.
26. Koda M, Okamoto K, Miyoshi Y, Kato S, Murawaki Y, Horie Y, Suou T, Kawasaki H. Combination therapy with transcatheter arterial embolization and percutaneous ethanol injection for advanced hepatocellular carcinoma. Hepato-Gastroenterol 1994;41:25–29.
27. Ito T, Urabe K, Shiraga K, Sakaguchi K, Higashi T, Hino N, Tsuji T. Retrospective analysis of multidisciplinary treatment for 534 hepatocellular carcinoma patients over a 12-year period. Int Med 1995;34:623–627.

Progress in Hepatology, Volume 3.
Hepatocellular Carcinoma.
M. Yamanaka, G. Toda and T. Tanaka, editors.

The usefulness of proton irradiation for hepatocellular carcinoma: present status and future prospects

Yasushi Matsuzaki[1], Toshiya Chiba[1], Junich Shoda[1], Naomi Tanaka[1], Toshiyuki Okumura[2], Hiroshi Tsuji[2] and Yasuyuki Akine[2]
[1]Division of Gastroenterology and Hepatology, Institute of Clinical Medicine, University of Tsukuba; and [2]Proton Medical Research Center, University of Tsukuba, Tsukuba, Ibaraki 305, Japan

Abstract. Proton beams are characterized with an excellent dose localization because of its Bragg-peak. We previously reported that a large dose of proton irradiation can be safely given to patients with hepatocellular carcinoma (HCC) complicated with liver cirrhosis. The aim of this study is to show the usefulness of proton therapy for HCC and clarify the role of this new therapy. Proton irradiation was given to 62 patients with 91 nodular HCC, who were considered either surgically or medically inoperable. Thirty-five out of the 62 patients with 53 lesions were treated with proton alone (monotherapy group). The remaining 27 patients with 38 lesions were treated with a combined therapy of proton irradiation and Lipiodol®-targeted chemotherapy (combination therapy group). A total dose of 75 Gy on average was given to them. Local control rates and survival rates were compared with those for 42 patients with HCC treated with Lipiodol®-targeted chemotherapy alone (l-TAI group) during the same period at the same institution. Both local control and survival rates for patients treated with proton therapy (monotherapy and combination therapy group) were significantly higher than those for l-TAI group. No patients treated with proton therapy experienced any serious adverse effects. Excellent quality of life (QOL) was maintained in all the patients treated with proton therapy during the follow-up periods. In conclusion, proton therapy is effective and safe in the treatment of HCC. Its striking advantages include very few side effects during the treatment as well as excellent QOL during and after the treatment. Furthermore, it could easily treat patients with serious complications and could irradiate deeply seated tumors.

Keywords: Bragg-peak, heavy ionized charged particle, hepatocellular carcinoma, proton beam, proton irradiation, QOL, radiation therapy.

Background

Primary hepatocellular carcinoma (HCC) is well recognized as one of the most malignant tumors in the Far East and Sub-Saharan Africa with a dismal prognosis [1,2]. Its prognosis is very poor and median survival is 1.6 months in untreated patients [3]. Recent progress in imaging techniques owing to the use of ultrasonography, angiography or CT scan has permitted earlier diagnosis of small HCC. Thus, the natural course of the patients with HCC < 3 cm is 90% at 1 year, 12% at 3 years with an average survival period of 20.7 months [4].

Recently, although surgery offers the best hope of cure for HCC, many patients

Address for correspondence: Yasushi Matsuzaki MD PhD, Assistant Professor, Division of Gastroenterology and Hepatology, Institute of Clinical Medicine, University of Tsukuba, 1-1-1 Tennodai, Tsukuba, Ibaraki 305, Japan. Tel./Fax: +81-298-53-3124.

have inoperable tumors at the time of presentation. The number of resectable cases is limited even for small HCC because of the unique clinicopathological characteristics of this carcinoma, including multifocality, early vascular invasions, or pre-existing advanced liver cirrhosis [5]. Alternative nonsurgical therapies such as transcatheter arterial embolization (TAE) [6—8], Lipiodol®-targeted chemotherapy [9,10], percutaneous ethanol injection therapy (PEIT) [11,12], radiotherapy, cryotherapy, hyperthermia or liver transplantation [13], have been introduced and proved to be successful to some extent, however, their anticancer effects are often insufficient to obtain local tumor control.

The role of radiation therapy in the treatment of HCC has been of limited use among recently developed therapeutic modalities. For the therapy of 11,397 cases with HCC during 2 years in Japan, the treatment was conducted with surgery in 33% (3,803 out of 11,379 cases), chemoembolization in 63.9% (6,518/10,193 cases), ethanol injection in 16.1% (1,586/9,896 cases), whereas radiation was used only in 0.8% (75/9,644 cases) [14].

Early attempts of radiation therapy for HCC have yielded disappointing results [15—18] because severe adverse effects on the liver as well as on other organs did not permit irradiation of sufficient quantity and duration. This conventional radiotherapy failed to obtain good local tumor control and subsequently led to poor outcome.

Moreover, many studies on the therapeutic efficacy including radiotherapy are difficult to compare with each other, since the study design, patients selection, or criteria of objective response are not uniform. Whether it is primary HCC or metastatic liver cancer and whether HCC is nodular, massive or diffuse type is also important for comparison.

A novel, powerful radiotherapy using proton beams (proton therapy), however, has recently been successful in treating various malignancies [19—25] except for

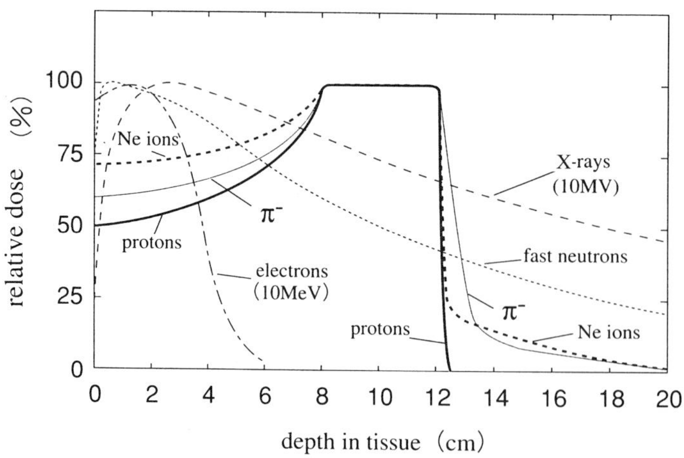

Fig. 1. Comparison of depth-dose curve of a proton beam with another radiation beam.

HCC. As shown in Fig. 1, the proton beam has Bragg-peak which can limit the distribution of the beams [22]. This results in both a marked reduction in the amount of radiation that reaches nontargeted areas and an increase in the amount of radiation hitting the targeted lesion.

In 1992, we preliminary reported that a large dose of proton irradiation can be safely administered to HCC patients with pre-existing cirrhosis [26]. Moreover, in 1994 and 1995, we reported that proton irradiation was a safe and effective therapeutic option in cases of HCC [27,28]. Here, we demonstrate the present status and the future prospects of the proton irradiation for HCC.

Clinical results of proton irradiation for HCC

Irradiation procedure of proton beam

Proton therapy was performed at the Proton Medical Research Center (PMRC) of University of Tsukuba in collaboration with the National Laboratory for High Energy Physics (KEK). The protons were provided by a booster synchrotron of KEK. Their energy was reduced from 500 MeV before use to 250 MeV.

For the planning of proton radiotherapy, we used the CT taken at sections of 5 to 10 mm in the lesion [29]. We performed automatic extraction of the body framework on the CT. Then, the targeted framework was input using a trackball. When the incident direction was determined, CT value electron density conversion was conducted on a line passing through the target in the incident direction, and a new file was prepared. Based on these data, the irradiated area, Bragg-peak formation and isodose line were planned.

By using a localized verify system, such setup errors were minimized to ±1 mm. The setup time was 5–10 min, and the actual exposure was 2–5 min. To avoid irradiation to lungs, a respiratory synchronized system was developed for tumors unable to remain stable due to respiration [30].

Based on the characteristics of protons, without using the multiple-field technique or moving-field therapy, the HCC lesion alone was selectively subjected to one-, two-, or three-field, lesion-fixed irradiation using a bolus (distribution adjuster of beam amount). Our policy for defining a target volume has been to add the smallest possible margins around the tumor volume; 5–10 mm of grossly normal tissue around the radiographically demonstrable tumor was usually included in the treatment volume. In those patients with single-node HCC, the irradiation was restricted to the margins around the target tumor. In case the tumors were multiple, all the targeted tumors were included in one radiated field.

The dose contour around the target volume was set at the prescribed 100% dose level. A relative biological effectiveness (RBE) value of 1.0 relative to ^{60}Co was used. One course of treatment consisted of daily fraction size ranging from 2.5 to 6.0 Gy (median 4.0 Gy) and the duration was 13–56 days (median 33 days). Total amount of radiation ranged from 50–87 Gy (median 72 Gy).

Treatment evaluation

Treatment evaluation was performed for a period of 3 weeks, every year from 1 to 5 years after completing the proton therapy.

Firstly, the reduction of the tumor size was estimated on CT as the product of the two largest perpendicular diameters. The tumor size reduction rate was calculated by tumor size and expressed as a percentage. Local tumor control meant no sign of regrowth or development of new lesions at the irradiated site.

The tumor response to the treatment was also judged according to serum α-fetoprotein (AFP) values. Routine liver function tests were performed 1 week after the therapy and monthly thereafter.

Quality of life (QOL) during and after proton therapy was estimated by the grade of performance status (PS) using the WHO handbook for reporting results of cancer treatment [31].

Tissue biopsy of the irradiated tumor was performed using a fine-diameter needle (21-G Majima needle®) under ultrasonography at 3 weeks after completing the proton therapy.

Patients

Our study was approved by the Ethical Committee of Tsukuba University. Patients were taken for informed consent and received proton beam radiotherapy (proton therapy) between January 1988 and January 1995.

Ninety-one lesions in 62 patients with single or multinodular tumors were treated altogether. They were selected from those who refused surgery or had unresectable HCC. The reasons of unresectability were multiple tumors, vessel invasions, complications with advanced cirrhosis or chronic renal failure and myelodysplastic syndrome. Also, those with insufficient accumulation of Lipiodol in the lesion of Lipiodol-targeted chemotherapy were included. All patients had accompanying liver cirrhosis graded as Child A (32 patients), Child B (17 patients) and Child C (13 patients). Three patients had portal invasion.

We performed nonrandomized controlled study of proton therapy for HCC. The 62 proton-treated patients with 91 HCC lesions were compared with 42 patients with 65 lesions treated with l-TAI alone during the same period of time, as a control, and the backgrounds did not differ among the groups.

We divided the patients treated with proton into two groups according to the mode of combined treatment, i.e., either by proton therapy only (monotherapy group) or by proton therapy combined with by Lipiodol®-targeted chemotherapy which resulted in insufficient accumulation of Lipiodol® into the tumors (combination therapy group). For the monotherapy group of 53 lesions in 35 patients Lipiodol®-targeted chemotherapy was not given because of advanced pre-existing liver cirrhosis, chronic renal failure, or myelodysplastic syndrome. On the other hand, 27 patients with 38 lesions in the combination group received proton therapy as additional treatment to Lipiodol®-targeted chemotherapy. As a control group, 42 patients with 65 lesions were treated by l-TAI only.

Tumor size ranged 1.0—10.0 cm among all the groups, average size was approximately 3.0 cm.

Reduction of tumor size and local tumor control

Figure 2 shows the tumor size reduction which means radiation effect. After 1 year, the reduction of tumor size was observed in 47 out of 50 lesions (94%) in monotherapy, 33 out of 35 lesions (94%) in combination therapy, compared with 36 out of 52 lesions (69%) in l-TAI group. After 2 years, size reduction was seen in 15 of 19 (79%) in monotherapy, 12 of 15 (80%) in combination therapy and 17 of 23 (74%) in l-TAI group. After 4 years, size reduction was seen in 3 of 3 (100%) in monotherapy, 3 of 3 (100%) in combination and 4 of 6 (67%) in l-TAI group.

By Kaplan-Meier's methods, cumulative local tumor control rate was significantly higher in the proton groups (Mono and Combi) than in the l-TAI group

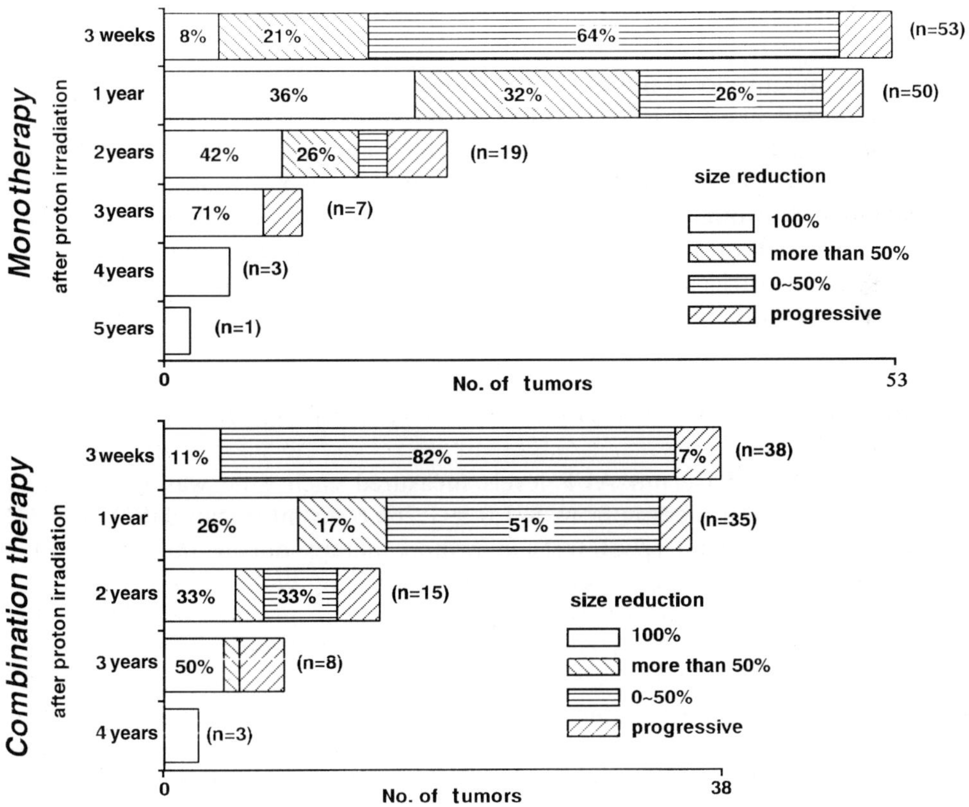

Fig. 2. Number of tumors with size reduction 3 weeks to 5 years after proton irradiation (monotherapy and combination therapy) in HCC cases.

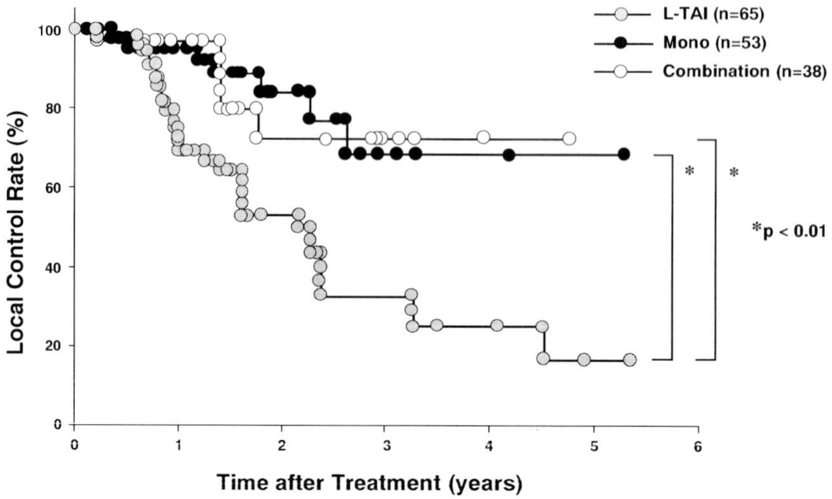

Fig. 3. Cumulative local tumor control rate after proton therapy and/or lipiodol targeted chemotherapy.

(Fig. 3). Cumulative local tumor control rates, at the end of the 1st year: 97% for both Mono and Combi, 70% for l-TAI group, at the end of the 3rd year: 69% for Mono, 73% for Combi, 33% for l-TAI group, and at the end of the 5th year, 69% for Mono, 17% for l-TAI. Figure 4 shows the demonstrable CT imaging before and after proton irradiation.

No patients died of the adverse effects of proton therapy but some died of liver cirrhosis such as variceal hemorrhage. Thus, even for the patients in handicapped condition, proton therapy was effective enough to reduce the size and to control the tumors.

Tumor marker

As shown in Fig. 5, serum AFP levels measured each time was significantly reduced after proton therapy from 571.0 ± 1,266.6 ng/ml (mean ± SD, n = 34) to 145.4 ± 346.3 ng/ml ($p<0.001$) in proton therapy during the period of 3 months.

Pathological changes

Follow-up biopsies 3 weeks after proton therapy did not show any viable cancer cells in 9 (75%) out of 12 lesions. In one patient with viable cancer cells, the tumor disappeared 5 weeks after biopsy. Hence, there was a discrepancy in the time lag between the reduction of tumor size and the improvement of histology. Therefore the effectiveness of the treatment should be judged both from the tumor size and histology or even devascularization of tumor on angiography. As is often

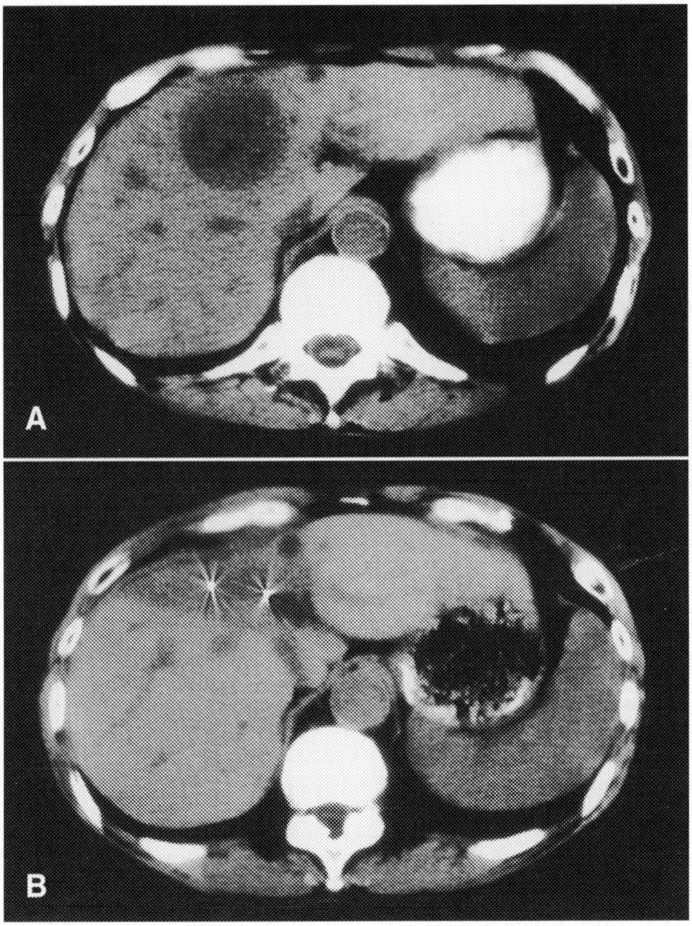

Fig. 4. X-ray CT images before (**A**) and 1 year after (**B**) proton therapy.

seen in the case of transcatheter arterial embolization, it is not infrequent that the content of the tumor is completely necrotic although tumor size on CT remained unchanged. This situation may exist in the irradiated cases with proton therapy.

Side effects

As shown in the Table 1, it is noteworthy that the incidences of side effects are very low in proton therapy. No patients experienced any serious adverse reactions. No clinical symptoms such as general fatigue, appetite loss and nausea were seen. Elevation of aspartate aminotransferase or alanine aminotransferase was observed twice more than the base line level up to 500 IU/l in 14 out of 62 patients (23%), which improved down to 12% at present. But these abnormalities recovered rapidly to normal level within 1—2 weeks during irradiation. Transient

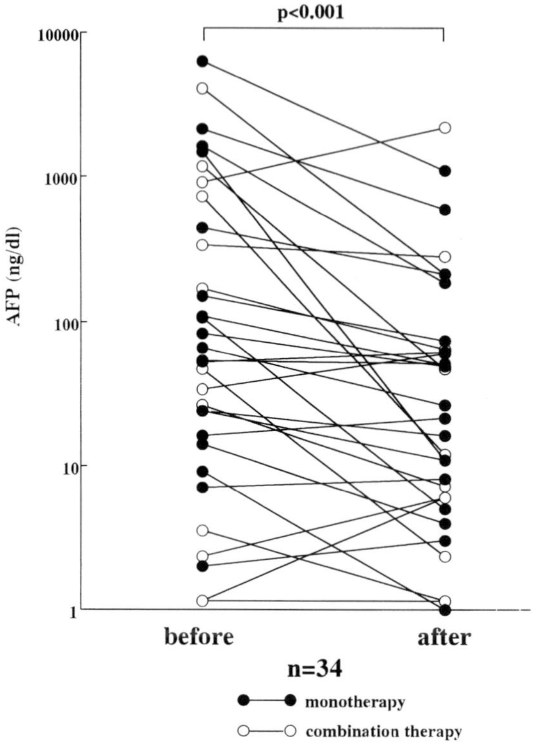

Fig. 5. Changes of AFP levels before and after proton therapy.

elevation of serum aminotransferase might have been caused due to local radiation hepatitis in the area by proton beam before reaching the target tumor.

Leukocytopenia ($<3{,}000/mm^3$) was seen in 24 out of 62 cases (39%), thrombopenia ($<5\times 10\ mm^3$) in 30%, and decreased hemoglobin (>2 g, more than base line value) in 3%. All these abnormalities recovered 2 weeks after irradiation. None of these patients have experienced any other serious side effects necessitating the discontinuation of the irradiation therapy.

Table 1. Side effects of proton irradiation for HCC.

Side effect	Mono cases (%)	Combination cases(%)
Fever ($>38°C$)	0/35 (0)	0/27 (0)
Abdominal pain	0/35 (0)	0/27 (0)
Pleural effusion	0/35 (0)	0/27 (0)
Elevation of transaminase	7/35 (20)	7/27 (26)
Elevation of T-Bil (>3.0 mg/dl)	3/35 (9)	4/27 (15)
Anemia ($>$Hb 2 g/dl)	1/35 (3)	1/27 (4)
Leukocytopenia ($<3{,}000/mm^3$)	10/35 (29)	14/27 (52)
Thrombocytopenia ($<5\times 10^4/mm^3$)	9/35 (26)	10/27 (37)

Performance status

Figure 6 shows the PS before and immediately after finishing the proton therapy. In 83.1% patients there was no change in PS in the Mono group, on the other hand in l-TAI group, 57.5% patients deteriorated in PS. All patients maintained their usual lifestyle, and there were no restrictions in physically strenuous activities during proton therapy. QOL was insured throughout the treatment period.

Long-term follow-up

Proton irradiated patients were followed more than 3 months up to 6 years. Survival rate was also significantly higher in the proton groups than in the l-TAI group during the follow-up period. Cumulative survival rates in three groups were as follows; at the end of the 2nd year, 86% for Mono, 92% for Combi, 59% for l-TAI, at the end of the 4th year, 67% for Mono, 81% for Combi, 36% for l-TAI (Fig. 7).

According to the liver function (Child-Pugh classification), we compared the cumulative survival rates among the three groups. In Child-Pugh A group, the Mono and Combi groups have significantly higher survival rates compared to the l-TAI groups. In Child-Pugh B and C, there was no statistically significant difference among the three groups.

In Child-Pugh A and B groups, the survival rate of the Combi and Mono groups are higher than that of the l-TAI group. Moreover, between Mono and

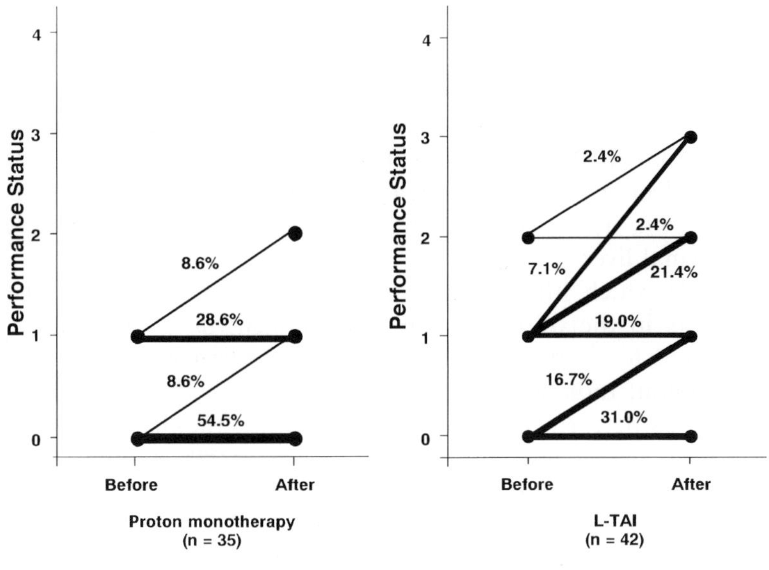

Fig. 6. Effects of proton or lipiodol targeted chemotherapy on performance status of patients with HCC.

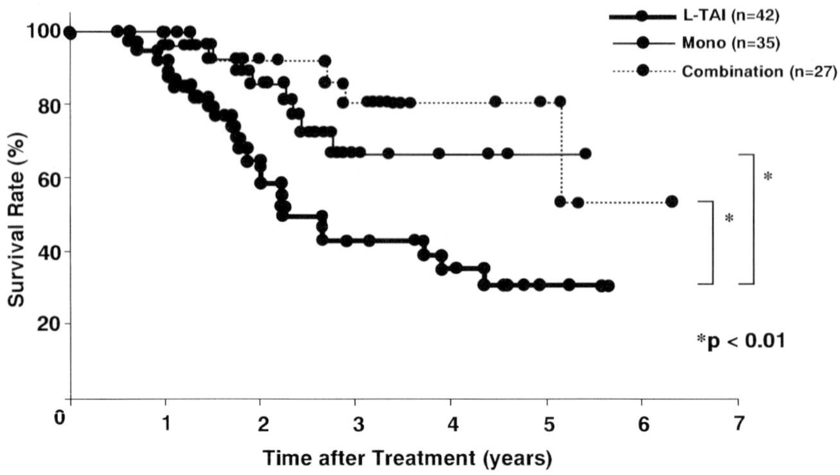

Fig. 7. Cumulative survival rate after proton therapy and/or lipiodol targeted chemotherapy.

Combi groups, the cumulative survival rate of Combi group is significantly higher than that of Mono group.

Discussion

Conventional external radiation for HCC

Major reasons for the limited usage of radiation therapy are attributable to the fact that radiation has not been capable of curing HCC, and that the tolerance of radiation of the normal liver is much lower than the tumoricidal dose. It has long been known that the tolerance dose of the whole normal liver is approximately in the range of 25—40 Gy [32—34]. Furthermore, more than 80% of HCC are coexisted with liver cirrhosis. Although the tolerance of the tissue of cirrhosis is not exactly known, it is speculated that cirrhotic liver can tolerate less irradiation than the normal liver.

Therefore, the obstacle which hindered the use of radiation therapy for the treatment of HCC exists in the difficulty that the sufficient dose of radiation beam should be delivered to the tumor, while the surrounding hepatic tissues are irradiated safely without radiation induced liver injury. On the other hand, whole liver irradiation was performed as early as 1940, when the demonstration of the tumor in the liver was technically difficult. It was mostly employed for the palliative care of the metastatic liver cancer.

Recently, as the imaging techniques such as angiography or CT scan progress in demonstrating the distinct localization of the tumor in the liver, whole or partial liver irradiation has been tried. There are some reports that the tumor regression with durable response is possible with an adequate dose of radiation. Ohto et al.

[35] demonstrated 39 patients with HCC using the linear accelerator. Over 25% of size reduction was observed in 90% of patients with < 5 cm in tumor size. In > 5 cm tumor in size, 58% patients showed over 50% size reduction. Recently, Matsuura et al. [36] reported 16 residual or recurrent HCC who were treated with radiation of $58 \sim 64$ Gy following TAE, 75% of local tumor control was gained at 6 months, 45% at 1 year, 45% at 2 years and 36% at 3 years.

In contrast to the reports mentioned above, Aoki et al. [37] showed that $50 \sim 70$ Gy of local irradiation caused 33% of partial response (PR) in seven cases with HCC, but all cases showed marked shrinkage of liver at autopsy. Histological examination revealed viable cancer cells in all cases. They concluded that local radiotherapy of $50 \sim 70$ Gy was not capable of curing HCC.

In summary, previous reports on conventional radiation therapy for HCC have shown disappointing results except for some successful reports [5,38–41]. It has been assumed that more than 50 Gy should be targeted for killing HCC cells [42]. However, those conventional approaches in which the whole liver is irradiated have caused radiation hepatitis and eventual hepatic failure, especially in patients complicated with cirrhosis. Therefore, sufficient irradiation of large doses to obtain effective antineoplastic effects for most cases of HCC have not been possible [40–42].

Present status of heavy charged particle therapy: powerful proton radiotherapy

Physical characteristics of proton

Proton is a particle which is produced by depriving electron from hydrogen atom. Hence, it is positively charged and weighs 1,836 times heavier than electron. Particles which are heavier than electron are called heavy particles; there are two kinds of heavy particles, charged and uncharged. Fast neutron is a heavy uncharged particle and proton, heavy ions (carbon, neon or argon), helium and negative pi-meson are the heavy charged particles.

Dose distribution of proton beam

Proton becomes an ionized beam with strong penetration power when it is accelerated to high energy by the accelerator. Along the path of a proton beam its positive charge interacts with the electron of atoms, which compose body tissue, resulting in ionization and excitation of the atoms until it finally looses energy and stops. Unlike the conventional radiation beam, the proton beam has a unique dose distribution. It has a peak area (Bragg-peak) where rapidly increasing doses are deposited at the end of the beam range defined with the particular beam energy [19–21,23] (Fig. 1). Therefore proton therapy has an advantage that a large dose of radiation can be focused only on the target, and the irradiation of surrounding nontumor tissues can be limited to as little as possible [19–23]. This is completely different from the photon (X-ray or gamma ray) which looses its energy exponentially with depth inside the tissue. This is the reason why the proton can be used to irradiate cancer selectively, avoiding normal tissues. Therefore proton therapy is one of the modes of external radiation therapy having a potential almost equivalent to surgery in terms of local cure of the lesion.

The distribution of the dose can be designed so as to conform to the requirements of the individual patients, i.e., Bragg-peak can be adjusted to targeted focus in width and depth according to the depth and the shape of tumor, so as to give the concentrated dose to the tumor [43].

Biological feature of a proton beam
Biological effect of a radiation beam depends on the linear energy transfer (LET), which is defined as the energy received by the surrounding tissue along the unit distance of the track of a charged particle. The RBE of the proton is $0.9 \sim 1.3$, which is almost equal to gamma ray. Thus, the feature of the proton for the treatment of cancer is that it has a suitable dose distribution (Bragg-peak) and an RBE equivalent to X- or gamma ray.

Circumstance of proton therapy
In 1938, Lawrence Berkley Laboratory (LBL) started the first heavy particle treatment by using fast neutron supplied from an accelerator designed for the physics laboratory. In 1954, they started irradiation of heavy charged particle, using the proton, followed by helium ion (1957) and heavier particles (1975).

In 1990, Loma Linda University set up a hospital-based proton beam treatment center for the first time, which was dedicated to medical service and research [44]. Currently, proton therapy is being carried out in 17 facilities in the world, and up to now over 16,000 patients have been treated. Proton therapy has been applied mainly for small lesions of the eye and the brain. About 46% of all proton treatment was for intracranial lesions (pituitary adenoma and arteriovenous misformation), 32% for eye cancer and 22% for mainly skull base and cervical spine sarcoma. It is noteworthy, especially, that 96—99% of 5 years local control was obtained for uveal melanoma [45].

On the basis of the above, excellent control rates of clinical trials, proton treatment became a field of increasing interest. However, few cases of the deep seated tumor in the abdomen or chest has been treated. In 1983, Tsukuba Proton Medical Center, University of Tsukuba, started proton irradiation for multisite malignancies in collaboration with KEK [46,47], and we began to try to treat HCC using proton irradiation.

Summary and future prospects

In summary, our study showed that proton irradiation is safe and effective for the nodular HCC in terms of tumor size reduction and excellent local tumor control was obtained during the observation period. Moreover, HCC patients treated with proton irradiation showed more excellent local tumor control as well as better survival and QOL, in comparison with l-TAI, which lasted for at least 5 years. This therapy is safe and has a special merit of excellent QOL during the treatment without any complaints. One of the striking advantages of this therapy is that it can treat patients with deep-seated tumors, those with serious complications, and or even with associated portal vein thrombus. Because of the excellent local tumor control, the determining factor for the survival is not affected by the proton irradiation but by the associated complications such as liver cirrhosis. Major limitation is solely that HCC should be nodular and not diffuse type.

New interest in the radiation therapy for HCC is growing recently, since irradiation itself has a potency of curing HCC. Much progress has been made over the past 10 years in the efforts to deliver a large amount of tumoricidal radiation dose to the tumor with acceptable complications. In the future, proton irradiation is another novel, effective and safe therapeutic option which can be applied as one of the therapies of curative intent. In fact, there is a wide variety of heterogeneity of the patients with varying degree of cirrhosis and HCC tumor itself. It is most important to choose the adequate treatment modality among many options, although there are arguments about the comparable efficacy between those treatments.

Today in Japan, where HCC is the third cause of death in man, unresectable tumor is treated most widely with chemoembolization or PEIT. If the unresectable tumors could be controlled for a long period by such nonsurgical treatment including radiation, survival rate and prognosis of the patient would largely depend on the underlying liver disease, management of which has been remarkably improved today, albeit the possibility of new recurrence from other focus due to multifocality of HCC.

In the future the efficacy of repeated treatment or combined therapy with other methods should be studied. Also the indication will be expanded for the liver metastasis especially of colon cancer after operation which is the major factor for the survival of this increasing disease.

Acknowledgements

This study was supported by research project grant-in-aid for scientific research No. 06670518 from the Ministry of Education, Science and Culture as well as University of Tsukuba Project Research.

The authors thank Professor Yuji Itai, Hirohiko Tsujii MD, for their radiological guidance, Mikio Doy MD, for his helpful liver histology, Professor Toshiaki Osuga, Yoshifumi Saito MD and Shinji Yoshiga MD, for their helpful suggestions and for preparing the manuscript.

Reference

1. Linsell DA, Higginson J. The geographic pathology of liver cell cancer. In: Cameron HM, Linsell DA, Warwich GP (ed) Liver Cancer. New York: Elsevier, 1976:1–16.

2. Beasley RP. Hepatitis B virus as the etiologic agent in hepatocellular carcinoma-epidemiologic considerations. Hepatology 1982;2(Suppl):21–26.
3. Okuda K, Ohtsuki T, Obata H, Tomimatsu M, Okazaki N, Hasegawa H, Nakajima Y, Ohnishi K. Natural history of hepatocellular carcinoma and prognosis in relation to treatment. Cancer 1985;56:918–928.
4. Ebara M, Ohto M, Shinagawa T, Sigiura N, Kimura K, Matsutani S, Morita M, Sasho H, Tsuchiya Y, Okuda K. Natural history of minute hepatocellular carcinoma smaller than three centimeters complicating cirrhosis: a study in 22 patients. Gastroenterology 1986;90:289–298.
5. Dusheiko GM, Hobbs KE, Dick R, Burroughs AK. Treatment of small hepatocellular carcinoma. Lancet 1992;340:285–288.
6. Nakamura H, Hashimoto T, Oi H, Sawada S. Transcatheter oily chemoembolization of hepatocellular carcinoma. Radiology 1989;170:783–786.
7. Ohishi H, Yoshimura H, Uchida H, Sakaguchi H, Yoshida T, Ohue S, Matsui T, Takaya A, Tsujii T. Transcatheter arterial embolization using iodized oil (Lipiodol®) mixed with an anticancer drug for the treatment of hepatocellular carcinoma. Cancer Chemother Pharmacol 1989;23 (Suppl):S33–S36.
8. Yamada R, Kishi K, Sonomura T, Tsuda M, Nomura S, Satoh M. Transcatheter arterial embolization in unresectable hepatocellular carcinoma. Cardiovasc Intervent Radiol 1990;13: 135–139.
9. Kuroda C, Sakurai M, Monden M, Marukawa T, Hosoki T, Tokunaga K, Wakasa K, Okamura J, Kozuka T. Limitation of transcatheter arterial chemoembolization using iodized oil for small hepatocellular carcinoma: a study in resected cases. Cancer 1991;67:81–86.
10. Novell JR, Dusheiko G, Markham NI, Reddy K, Dick R, Hobbs KE. Selective regional chemotherapy of unresectable hepatic tumors using lipiodol. Hepatic Pancreatic Biliary 1991; 4:223–236.
11. Sheu JC, Huang GT, Chen DS, Sung JL, Yang PM, Wei TC, Lai MY, Su CT, Tsang YM, Hsu HC, Su IJ, Wu TT, Lin JT, Chuang CN. Small hepatocellular carcinoma: intratumor ethanol treatment using new needle and guidance systems. Radiology 1987;163:43–48.
12. Tanikawa K. Nonsurgical treatment of hepatocellular-carcinoma. Jpn J Gastroenterol Surgery 1990;23:2492–2496.
13. Venook AP. Treatment of hepatocellular carcinoma: too many options? J Clin Oncol 1994;12:1323–1334.
14. Liver Cancer Study Group of Japan. Survey and follow-up study of primary liver cancer in Japan, Report 11. Acta Hepatologica Japonica 1994;14:208–218.
15. Geddes E, Falkson G. Malignant hepatoma in the Bantu. Cancer 1970;25:1271–1278.
16. Falkson G. Therapeutic approaches to hepatoma. Cancer Treat Rev 1975;2:73–76.
17. Ong G, Chan P. Primary carcinoma of the liver. Surg Gynecol Obstet 1976;143:31–38.
18. Cochrane AMG, Murray-Lyon IM, Brinkley DM, Williams R. Quadruple chemotherapy versus radiotherapy in treatment of primary hepatocellular carcinoma. Cancer 1977;40:609–661.
19. Graffman S, Jung B. Clinical trials in radiotherapy and the merits of high energy protons. Acta Radiol 1970;9:1–23.
20. Raju MR, Phillips TL. The potential for heavy particle radiation therapy. LA-6588-MS. Los Alamos, UC-48, 1977, 1–52.
21. Suit HD, Goitein M, Tepper JE, Verhey L. Clinical experience and expectation with protons and heavy ions. Int J Radiat Oncol Biol Phys 1977;3:115–125.
22. Suit HD, Goitein M. Rationale for use of charged-particle and fast-neutron beams in radiation therapy. In: Meyn RE, Withers HR (eds) Radiation Biology in Cancer Research. New York: Raven Press, 1980:547–565.
23. Suit HD, Goitein M, Munzenrider J, Verhey L, Blitzer P, Gragoudas E, Koehler AM, Urie M, Gentry R, Shipley W, Urano M, Duttenhaver J, Wagner M. Evaluation of the clinical applicability of proton beams in definitive fractionated radiation therapy. Int J Radiat Oncol Biol Phys 1982;8:2199–2205.

24. Chuvilo IV, Goldin LL, Khoroshkov VS, Blokhin SE, Breyev VM, Vorontsov IA, Elmolayev VV, Kleinbock YA, Lomakin MI, Lomanov MF, Medved VY, Miliokhin NA, Narinsky VM, Pavlonsky LM, Shimchuck GG. ITEP synchrotron proton beam in radiotherapy. Int J Radiat Oncol Biol Phys 1984;10:185–195.
25. Suit HD, Goitein M, Munzenrider L, Verhey L, Urie M, Gragoudas E, Koehler A, Gottschalk B, Sisterson J, Tatsuzaki H, Miralbell R. Increased efficacy of radiation therapy by use of proton beam. Strahlenther Onkol 1990;166:40–44.
26. Tanaka N, Matsuzaki Y, Chuugannji Y, Osuga T, Kuramoto K, Tsujii H. Proton irradiation for hepatocellular carcinoma. The Lancet 1992;Nov.28:1358.
27. Matsuzaki Y, Osuga T, Saito Y, Chugannji Y, Tanaka N, Shoda J, Tsuji H, Tsujii H. A new, effective and safe therapeutic option using proton irradiation for hepatocellular carcinoma. Gastroenterology 1994;106:1032–1041.
28. Matsuzaki Y, Osuga T, Chiba T, Saito Y, Tanaka N, Itai Y, Tsujii H. New, effective treatment using proton irradiation for unresectable hepatocellular carcinoma. Int Med 1995;34:302–304.
29. Tsujii H, Inada T, Maruhashi A, Hayakawa Y, Tsuji H, Ohara K, Akisada M, Kitagawa T. Field localization and verification system for proton beam radiotherapy in deep-seated tumors. Nippon Acta Radiologica 1989;49:622–629.
30. Ohara K, Okumura T, Akisada M, Inada T, Mori T, Yokota Y, Calaguas MJB. Irradiation synchronized respiration gate. Int J Radiat Oncol Biol Phys 1989;17:853–857.
31. WHO handbook for reporting results of cancer treatment. WHO offset publication No. 48. WHO Geneva, 1979.
32. Ingold JA, Reed GB, Kaplan HS, Bagshaw MA. Radiation hepatitis. Am J Roentgenol 1965; 93:200–208.
33. Austin-Seymour NM, Chen GTY, Castro JR, Saunders WM, Pitluck S, Woodruff KH and Kessler M. Dose volume histogram analysis of liver radiation tolerance. Int J Radiat Oncol Biol Phys 1986;12:31–35.
34. Jirtle RL, Anscher MS, Alati T. Radiation sensitivity of the liver. Adv Radiat Biol 1990;14: 269–311.
35. Ohto M, Ebara M, Yoshikama M, Okuda K. Radiation therapy and percutaneous ethanol injection for the treatment of hepatocellular carcinoma. In: Neoplasms of the liver. Tokyo, Md: Springer-Verlag, 1987:335–341.
36. Matsuura M, Ishikawa A, Nakajima N, Itoh K, Matsumoto M. Radical radiation therapy for hepatocellular carcinoma. Nippon Acta Radiologica 1994;54:628–635.
37. Aoki K, Okaaki N, Okada S, Nose H, Yoshimori M, Akine Y, Egawa S, Sakamoto M, and Hirohashi S. Radiotherapy for hepatocellular carcinoma: clinicopathological study of seven autopsy cases. Hepatogastroenterology 1994;41:427–431.
38. Phillips R, Murikami K. Primary neoplasms of the liver. Cancer 1960;13:714–720.
39. Yu LY, Yu EX, Zheng P, Liu F, Gao LR, Hu AB, Zhang J, Liang W, Sing M, Zhu F. Radiotherapy of 217 patients with primary hepatocellular carcinoma (PHC). Excerpta Med Int Congr Ser 1981;542:286–293.
40. Ingold JA, Reed GB, Kaplan HS, Bagshaw MA. Radiation hepatitis. Am J Roentgenol Radium Ther Nucl Med 1965;93:200–208.
41. Lewin K, Millis RR. Human radiation hepatitis. Arch Pathol 1973;96:21–26.
42. El-Domeiri AA, Huvos AG, Goldsmith HS, Foote FW. Primary malignant tumors of the liver. Cancer 1971;27:7–11.
43. Kanai T, Kawachi K, Matsuzawa H, Inada T. Three-dimensional beam scanning for proton therapy. Nuclear Instr Meth 1983;214:491–496.
44. Slater JM, Miller DW, Archambeau JO. Development of a hospital-based proton beam treatment center. Int J Radiat Oncol Biol Phys 1988;14:761–775.
45. Suit H, Urie M. Proton beams in radiation therapy. J Natl Cancer Inst 1992;84:155–164.
46. Particle Radiation Medical Science Center, University of Tsukuba. Collected papers of PARMS (1980–1989) 1990;1–806.

47. Tsujii H, Tsuji H, Inada T, Maruhashi A, Hayakawa Y, Takada Y, Tada J, Fukumoto S, Tatsuzaki H, Ohhara K, Kitagawa T. Clinical results of fractionated proton therapy. Int J Radiat Oncol Biol Phys 1992;25:49–60.

Progress in Hepatology, Volume 3.
Hepatocellular Carcinoma.
M. Yamanaka, G. Toda and T. Tanaka, editors.

Gene therapy for hepatic tumors — micro-metastasis of colon carcinoma: a review in 1996

Yasushi Shiratori[1], Fumihiko Kanai[1], Yoko Hikiba[2], Hiroshi Moriyama[3], Hirofumi Hamada[4], Torao Tanaka[1], Keng-Hsin Lan[1], Makoto Ohashi[1], Masayuki Matsumura[2], Ken-ichi Okano[2], Makoto Naito[3] and Masao Omata[1]
[1]Department of Internal Medicine (II), Faculty of Medicine, University of Tokyo, Tokyo; [2]Division of Gastroenterology and Hepatology, Institute of Adult Disease, Asahi Life Foundation, Tokyo; [3]2nd Department of Pathology, Niigata University School of Medicine, Niigata-shi; [4]Department of Molecular Biotherapy Research, Cancer Chemotherapy Center, Cancer Institute, Japanese Foundation for Cancer Research, Tokyo, Japan

Keywords: adenovirus vector, cytokine gene therapy, gene therapy, gene transfer, hepatic metastasis of colon carcinoma, immunomodulation, interleukin-2, pit cells.

Introduction

Recent annual analysis reported from the Ministry of Health and Welfare indicated an increased number of patients with colon carcinoma the last 10—20 years in Japan. Colon carcinoma at an early stage is completely removed by surgery only, but its hepatic metastasis often hinders complete removal of tumor tissues from the body. As blood streams from the intestine to the liver, tumor cells invaded into the vascular lumen at the intestine are easily migrated to the liver and are easily trapped in the hepatic sinusoidal space, where tumor cells attach to the sinusoidal endothelial cells, invade, proliferate and establish metastatic foci. Recently, immunomodulation therapy for cancer has been proposed and applied to clinical trials. However, the immunomodulation therapy using recombinant cytokine proteins has not been satisfactory, as there are many serious side effects of cytokines. Various gene therapies for patients with metabolic deficient diseases have been developed and are recently used clinically, also several types of gene therapy have also been developed and used for cancer treatment. During these last 10 years, various functions of hepatic sinusoidal cells have been extensively studied, and functions of pit cells, liver-associated lymphocytes, have been clarified. In this chapter, gene therapy for hepatic metastasis of colon carcinoma by the modulation of hepatic sinusoidal cell function will be described comprehensively.

Address for correspondence: Yasushi Shiratori MD, Department of Internal Medicine (II), Faculty of Medicine, University of Tokyo, 7-3-1 Hongo, Bunkyo-ku, Tokyo 113, Japan. Tel.: +81-3-3815-5411. Fax: +81-3-3814-0021.

Cancer gene therapy in the liver

Strategies

The design of new treatment for cancer and genetic diseases consists of three strategies [1–4]: intervention of gene, transducted target cells and gene delivery system (Table 1).

Adequate molecular intervention

There are several proposals for selection of gene intervention for cancer gene therapy. Firstly, it should involve the identification of the gene type of molecular intervention that is appropriate, such as (a) replacement of mutant gene/tumor suppressor gene, (b) addition of DNA sequences expressing specific antisense transcript, (c) addition of suicide genes (G-DEPT), and (d) the insertion of sequence coding for toxins.

Methodology of gene insertion

A variety of methods can be used to increase the efficacy of DNA uptake by the cells, and the procedure can be mainly divided into three methods; (a) biological, (b) chemical and (c) physiological techniques (Table 2). Among these techniques, viral vectors are the most efficient means for the transfer of genes into target cells and are, therefore, preferred over physical methods.

Targeted cells by gene therapy

There are two notions for cancer gene therapy. Firstly, tumor cells are main tar-

Table 1. Strategy for gene therapy.

a) Intervention of gene
Tumor suppressor gene
GDEPT
Toxin
Immune response
b) Target cells (the cells to be transducted)
Tumor cell
Lymphocyte
Fibroblast
Hepatocyte
Keratinocyte
Myocyte
c) Delivery of gene
In vivo, ex vivo
Local, systemic
Receptor-targeted

Table 2. Gene insertion procedure.

a) Biological techniques
Retrovirus
Adenovirus
Parvovirus
Herpes simplex virus
b) Chemical techniques
Calcium phosphate
Liposomes
Asialo glycoprotein
c) Physical techniques
Direct injection
Microinjection
Electroporation

gets for the gene transduction, and secondly, expression of transducted gene may induce cytotoxicity to tumor cells in itself or induce sensitivity against several types of chain-terminator drug or cytotoxic lymphocytes. In addition to the gene therapy directed to the targeted tumor cell in itself, gene-directed immunotherapeutic strategies are based on the knowledge of host-tumor immune reaction. In this strategy, there are several proposals concerning inserting gene sequences; i.e. tumor-specific or tumor-associated antigens, MHC antigens or cytokines such as interleukin-2 (IL-2), interferon-r (INN) and tumor necrosis factor (TNF).

Rout of gene transduction

There are several procedures for the route of gene transduction. New genes may be delivered to cells (a) in vivo or ex vivo, (b) locally or systemically, and (c) the cell type to be targeted should be carefully defined. In an ex vivo gene transduction, after isolation of the cells from the organs obtained by surgery, the cells were cultured and were transfected in vitro with gene vector for the gene insertion. Subsequently, these transfected cells were then placed back in vivo into an appropriate place (i.e., spleen). In an in vivo gene transduction, gene transduction into tumor cells should be efficiently performed, but the specific delivery of the gene into the tumor cells remains unresolved when administered systemically. Instead, direct injection of gene vector into tumor mass was conducted. Hitherto, local delivery may be an effective way of treating a specific organ. To circumvent this pitfall of specific delivery of the gene into the tumor cells in vivo, tumor specific promotor (α-feto protein (AFP) promotor, carcinoembryonic antigen (CEA) promotor, etc) could be used for an enhanced expression of the transfected genes for specific expression of the gene in tumor cells exclusively.

Gene delivery into the liver

The development of strategies for gene therapy in the liver is a challenging task because the liver is involved in the manifestation of numerous genetic diseases and in malignant diseases. Hitherto, most of the available techniques for gene transfer were applied to hepatocytes ex vivo. Retroviral and adenoviral vectors have been studied with regard to hepatocyte-directed gene transfer in vivo and in vitro [5—7]. Attempts to retransplant retrovirally transduced hepatocytes back to patients was performed, but have shown the limit of the ex vivo approach.

The obvious alternative would be the development of suitable techniques for gene transfer in vivo using adenovirus vector; the comparative data using adenovirus or retrovirus vector are summarized in Table 3. Hepatocytes can be targets for clinical adenovirus infection, because the respiratory epithelium and the liver share the same embryonic origin. In fact, previous studies revealed that the adult liver could be a target for in vivo adenovirus-mediated gene transfer. The merits of adenovirus vector system are summarized in Table 4, i.e., organ specificity (hepatocytes), extent of expression, chronicity of expression and safety of recombinant adenovirus vector. In our previous studies, we have also demonstrated this notion using in vivo injection of adenovirus vector encoding an *Escherichia coli* lac Z gene in mice, indicating that an expression of lac Z gene was demonstrated in the liver only, but not in other organs.

Cytokine gene therapy for cancer

Cytokine gene therapy for cancer is one of four notions described previously (Table 5), i.e., genetic immunomodulation (insertion of a cytokine gene into tumor cells, in situ injection of plasmid carrying an HLA gene into a tumor mass that is negative for the injected HLA gene), virus-directed enzyme prodrug therapy (insertion of a suicide gene into tumor cells in situ with subsequent activation of the suicide mechanism) and gene replacement therapy (the use of tumor suppressor genes and/or antioncogene) and protection of host cells from anticancer drugs (the use of a multidrug resistant (MDR) gene to protect bone marrow cells or normal cells/tissues to allow higher-dose chemotherapy).

Strategy of the recent antitumor gene therapy of genetic immunomodulation is to use the vector of genes encoding several types of cytokines which induce and/

Table 3. Comparative data of adenovirus vector vs. retrovirus vector for gene transfer.

	Adenovirus	Retrovirus
Size of the trnsferred gene	7.5 kbp	8 kbp
Titer	10^{11}—10^{12} cfu/ml	10^{6}—10^{8} cfu/ml
Duration of expression	transient	indefinite
Expression level	high	low
Repeated administration	hampered by immune response	
Liver-directed gene therapy	yes	no
Risk	inflammatory response	insertional mutagenesis

Table 4. Adenovirus vector for gene therapy.

a) Organ specificity
   hepatocytes
b) Extent of expression
   high titer
c) Chronicity of expression
   turnover of hepatocytes
d) Safety of replication deficient recombinant virus
   adenovirus vector

or enhance cytotoxic T cell activity [8–10]. An application of these cytokines had already been shown to be a promising method in some cancer treatment using recombinant cytokines. However, various severe problems were resulting from the requirement to apply systemically high doses of the respective cytokines, since an application of therapeutically effective concentrations of biological active mediators is often accompanied by serious toxic side effects. Nowadays, these problems may be partly circumvented by "tumor cell targeted cytokine gene therapy": the tumor cells, that are genetically engineered to produce a given cytokine in vitro and/or upon injection into mice in vivo, provide a locally enhanced cytokine production from the transfected cells. This makes use of a more physiological mode of action of the cytokine to eventually chemotactically attract effector cells, and subsequently induce a tumor-specific immune response. Additionally, when the tumor cells were used as target of transfected genes, the source for the cytokine production is eliminated upon destruction of the tumor cells.

In addition to this "tumor cell targeted cytokine gene therapy" protocol, the cell type engineered to produce the cytokine is also crucial in the gene immunomodulation therapy, and the transfection of pleiotropic cytokine genes into the immune cells of the host in addition to tumor cells is proposed, Even in this type of gene therapy, the antitumor response can be enhanced by cytotoxic T cells and macrophages which can in turn be induced by an expression of appropriate

Table 5. Gene therapy for cancer.

a) Genetic immunomodulation
   cytokine gene
   HLA gene
b) Drug targeting
   virally directed enzyme prodrug therapy
   suicide gene – thymidine kinase (GCV)
   cytosine deaminase (5-FC)
c) Gene replacement
   tumor suppressor gene
   p53, RB, WT1, NF1, E-cadherin, nm23, JE/MCP1
   GCF, rap1A
d) Normal tissue protection
   MDR 1

cytokines by the cells. The best characterized model so far has been the transfection of the TNF gene into tumor-infiltrating lymphocytes (TIL) [11].

Cytokine gene therapy for liver tumors

Hepatic sinusoid unit

Liver lobule consists of parenchymal cells and hepatic sinusoidal cells such as Kupffer cells, peri-sinusoidal cells (fat-storing cells, lipocytes), hepatic sinusoidal endothelial cells, and pit cells (Fig. 1). Pit cells, organ-associated NK cells, are located in the hepatic sinusoid and ultrastructural features of these cells are similar to large granular lymphocytes (LGL) [12–17]. Previous studies including ours revealed that an administration of biological response modifier (BRM) increases the number of hepatic LGL and enhances their NK activity. In association with an increase in the number of pit cells and their NK activities, the formation of experimental hepatic metastasis of tumor cells was found to be reduced. Large granular lymphocytes (LGL), the morphological phenotype of natural killer (NK) cells, liver-associated LGL, and pit cells are of great interest because of their possible role in the immune surveillance and local immunological events [18,19]. These cells exert their cytotoxic activity against tumor cells, and may play an important role in the immune surveillance system in the liver even in a normal physiological state.

Immunomodulating gene therapy in the liver

Since liver-associated lymphocytes already exist in the liver, there may be a notion that specific delivery of cytokine genes into the liver might attract and activate neighboring lymphocytes and NK cells in the liver. Adenovirus vector

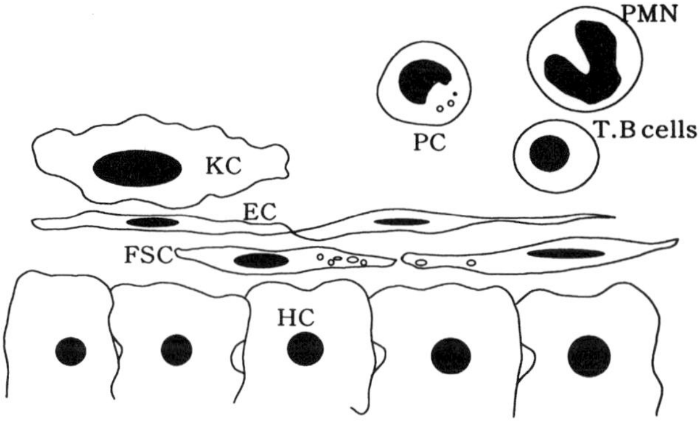

Fig. 1. Scheme of hepatic sinusoid. KC: Kupffer cells, EC: Endothelial cells, FSC: Fat-storing cells, PC: Perisinusoidal cells, HC: Hepatocytes, PMN: Polymorphonuclear cells, T.B cells: T cells, B cells (lymphocytes), PC: Pit cells.

is known to be specifically and efficiently targeted into the liver, especially in hepatocytes [5—7]. Thus, cytokines for enhanced NK activity encoded in adenovirus vector might provide a new strategy for enhanced immune surveillance system in the liver.

IL-2 is a growth factor that stimulates the proliferation of cytotoxic T cells, NK cells and LAK cells, all of which can participate in the antitumor response. In the mouse, systemic administration of IL-2 induces the expansion and long-term persistence of adoptively transferred tumor-specific T cells. However, systemic administration of cytokine IL-2 into experimental animals has been used but with an increased frequency of various adverse events. Since locally secreted cytokines were also able to influence the generation of antitumor immune responses with minor adverse effects, adenoviral vector could be used to introduce the IL-2 gene into the cells, such as malignant cells, immune competent cells, or normal tissues. Local secretion of IL-2 abrogated the tumorigenicity of the cytokine-producing malignant cells. By using the host immune system, the cells that were accumulated in some tumors, probably as a part of an immune attack on the tumor (tumor-infiltrating lymphocytes, TIL) via antitumor functions. Thus, an induction of paracrine antitumor immunoreactivity is modified to express potentially the gene therapy for cancer.

Experimental model of gene therapy for hepatic micrometastasis of colon carcinoma

IL-2 is known to enhance activity of NK cells, cytotoxic T cells and LAK cells [20,21]. Pit cells are located in the hepatic sinusoid and constitute organ-associated NK cells contributing to the immune surveillance in the liver. These cells are found to play an important role in the tumor defence system in the liver. Since pit cells show characteristic features of NK cells that could be activated by IL-2, the present study has been conducted to introduce the transduction of IL-2 gene into hepatocytes using adenovirus vector to produce IL-2 which might enhance NK activity of pit cells in the neighborhood, leading to inhibition of hepatic metastasis of colon carcinoma in vivo. Experimental model of immunomodulating gene therapy for hepatic metastasis of colon carcinoma was established using following vectors and tumor cell line.

Experimental animals. Male, SPF C57BL6 mice at the age of 8 weeks were used.

Hepatic metastasis of colon carcinoma. Hepatic metastasis of colon carcinoma was established by injection of colon 38 tumor cells into the superior mesenteric vein of the mice. Evaluation of hepatic metastasis was made 28 days after inoculation of tumor cells.

Vector. The recombinant adenovirus vector (Adex1CAmIL2) was constructed by inserting the expression unit composed of CAG promotor (cytomegalovirus enhancer plus chicken β-actin promotor), murine IL-2 cDNA and rabbit β-globin polyadenylation signal. After administration of Adex1CAmIL2 in vivo, expression of mIL-2 in hepatocytes was analyzed by immunostaining, northern blotting analysis, and in situ hybridization technique.

Discussion and Conclusion

Murine colon 38 adenocarcinoma, dimethylhydrazine-induced colon carcinoma, is known to be sensitive to lymphokine-activating killer cells or tumor-infiltrating lymphocytes (TIL) in combination with IL-2.

IL-2 is a growth factor of LGL/NK cells, and is known to be a potent stimulator for cytotoxic T lymphocytes. Previous study revealed that an enhancement of cell-mediated cytotoxicity was observed after 6-h stimulation of IL-2 in vitro, and that this enhancement was more significant after 24—72 h of culture. However, previous study revealed that pathological and toxicities induced by repeated intravenous or intraperitoneal injection of recombinant IL-2 have been reported; IL-2 administration may lead to the result of observed damage of the endothelial lining cells especially [13].

Recent study revealed that nonadherent, nonparenchymal liver cells have been reported to exert cytotoxicity against Yac 1 cells [15]. NK activity has been attributed to the cells having a morphology of LGL [20,21]. Previous study revealed that BRM administration showed a 4- to 6-fold increase in the number of pit cells [15]. In the previous study, IL-2 mRNA expression was found to be enhanced in the spleen after administration of BRM, but was demonstrated by only small amount in the liver [22]. The enhanced production of cytokine IL-2 from the spleen might be transmitted to the liver via the portal vein.

Bouwens et al. demonstrated that an accumulation of LGL and Kupffer cells in the liver of rats treated with continuous infusion of IL-2 [13]. In addition, previous study revealed that systemic administration of IL-2 showed a mild inhibitory effect of hepatic metastasis of colon carcinoma (unpublished observation).

Thus, it is of great interest for the potential immunotherapeutic treatment of liver metastasis with IL-2, and local treatment of IL-2 should be performed to reduce the serious side effects of IL-2. In these circumstances, IL-2 gene transduction using adenovirus vector may be one of the notions. IL-2 production from the transfected cells made cytotoxic T lymphocytes more potent in the liver in vivo. In these cases, systemic IL-2 concentration in serum was relatively low, but local concentration of IL-2 in the liver might be much higher.

Since local production of IL-2 may be important, the present study was conducted to use adenovirus vector to express the transducted cytokine gene in the liver. Although the number of hepatocytes transfected by Adex1CAmIL2 occupied only 2—3% of total hepatocytes, IL-2 production from the transfected hepatocytes renders neighboring lymphocytes activate and cytotoxic (enhancing NK activity). Thus, the number of hepatic metastasis of colon tumor cells was decreased in the liver when receiving Adex1CAmIL2. Thus, inhibition of hepatic metastasis of colon 38 adenocarcinoma was conducted by adoptive immunogene

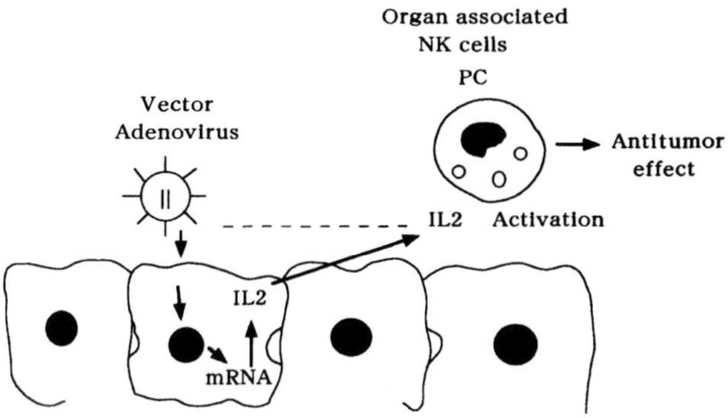

Fig. 2. Gene therapy for hepatic metastasis of colon carcinoma (scheme of experiment).

therapy of cancer.

From this study, the gene transduction using adenovirus was demonstrated in hepatocytes only, and local expression and production of IL-2 in hepatocytes enhance NK activity of neighboring liver-associated lymphocytes (pit cells), which subsequently exert their effort to induce cytotoxicity against tumor cells (Fig. 2). Thus, the number of hepatic metastasis was reduced in the mice after an administration of Adex1CAmIL2. This gene therapy is only effective within 7 days after tumor cell inoculation, during which the size of tumor foci remains small. This procedure may be clinically useful for inhibition of hepatic metastasis of colon carcinoma by enhancing activity of liver associated lymphocytes, pit cells. In addition to these notions, the gene therapy for specific targeting and adequate switch on-off system might provide further progression in modulating gene therapy in vivo.

References

1. Strauss M. Liver-directed gene therapy: prospective and problems. Gen Therapy 1994;1:156–164.
2. Li Q, Kay MA, Finegold M, Stratford-Perricaudet LD, Woo SLC. Assessment of recombinant adenoviral vectors for hepatic gene therapy. Hum Gene Therapy 1993;4:403–409.
3. Gutierrez AA, Lemoine NR, Sikora K. Gene therapy for cancer. Lancet 1992;339:715–721.
4. Gore ME, Collins MK. Gene therapy for cancer. Eur J Cancer 1994;30A:1047–1049.
5. Jaffe HA, Danel C, Longenecker G, Metzger M, Setoguchi Y, Rosenfeld MA et al. Adenovirus-mediated in vivo gene transfer and expression in normal rat liver. Nat Genet 1992;1:372–378.
6. Kass-Eisler A, Falck-Pedersen E, Elfenbein DH, Alvira M, Buttrick PM, Leinwand LA. The impact of developmental stage, route of administration and the immune system on adenovirus-mediated gene transfer. Gene Therapy 1994;1:395–402.
7. Kozarsky K, Wilson JM. Gene therapy: adenovirus vectors. Current Opinion in Genetics and Development 1993;3:499–503.
8. Chen SS, Chen XHL, Wang Y, Kosai KI, Finegold MJ, Rich SS, Woo SLC. Combination gene therapy for liver metastasis of colon carcinoma in vivo. Proc Natl Acad Sci USA 1995;92:2577–2581.

9. Nakamura Y, Wakimoto H, Abe J, Kanegae Y, Saito I, Aoyagi M, Hirakawa K, Hamada H. Adoptive immunotherapy with murine tumor-specific T lymphocytes engineered to secrete interleukin 2. Cancer Res 1994;54:5757–5760.
10. Gansbacher B, Zier K, Daniels B, Cronin K, Bannerji R, Gilboa E. Interleukin 2 gene transfer into tumor cells abrogates tumorigenicity and induces protective immunity. J Exp Med 1990; 172:1217–1224.
11. Blankenstein T, Qin Z, Uberla K, Muller W, Rosen H, Volk HD, Diamanstein T. Tumor suppression after tumor cell-targeted tumor necrosis factor alpha gene transfer. J Exp Med 1991;173: 1047–1052.
12. Bouwen L, Wisse E. Immuno-electron microscopic characterization of large granular lymphocytes (natural killer cells) from rat liver. Eur J Immunol 1987;17:1423–1428.
13. Bouwen L, Marinelli A, Kuppen PJK, Eggermont AMM, van de Velde CJH, Wisse E. Electron microscopic observations on the accumulation of large granular lymphocytes (Pit cells) and Kupffer cells in the liver of rats treated with continuous infusion of interleukin-2. Hepatology 1990;12:1365–1370.
14. Enzan H, Hiroi M, Saibara T, Onishi S, Yamamoto Y, Yamamoto H, Hara H. Immunoelectron microscopic identification of asialo-GM1-positive cells in adult rat liver. Virchows Archiv B Cell Pathol 1991;60:389–398.
15. Shiratori Y, Nakata R, Okano K, Komatsu Y, Shiina S, Kawase T, Sugimoto T et al. Inhibition of hepatic metastasis of colon carcinoma by asialo GM1-positive cells in the liver. Hepatology 1992;16:469–478.
16. Vanderkerken K, Bouwens L, Wisse E. Characterization of a phenotypically and functionally distinct subset of large granular lymphocytes (Pit cells) in rat liver sinusoids. Hepatology 1990; 12:70–75.
17. Shiratori Y, Tanaka M, Kawase T, Shiina S, Komatsu Y, Omata M. Quantification of sinusoidal cell function in vivo. Semin Liver Dis 1993;13:39–49.
18. Zarcone D, Prasthofer EF, Malavasi F, Pistoia V, LoBuglio AF, Grossi CE. Ultrastructural analysis of human natural killer cell activation. Blood 1987;69:1725–1736.
19. Wiltrout RH, Herberman RB, Zhang SR, Chirigos MA, Ortaldo JR, Green KM, Talmadge JE. Role of organ-associated NK cells in decreased formation of experimental metastases in lung and liver. J Immunol 1985;134:4267–4275.
20. Cohen SA, Salazar D, von Muenchhausen W, Werne-Wasik M, Nolan JP. Natural antitumor defense system of the murine liver. J Leukoc Biol 1985;37:559–569.
21. Trinchieri G, Ferussia B. Human natural killer cells: biologic and pathologic aspects. Lab Invest 1984;50:489–513.
22. Shiratori Y, Kawase T, Nakata R, Tanaka M, Hikiba Y, Okano K, Matsumura M et al. Effect of splenectomy on hepatic metastasis of colon carcinoma and natural killer activity in the liver. Dig Dis Sci 1995;40:2398–2406.

Progress in Hepatology, Volume 3.
Hepatocellular Carcinoma.
M. Yamanaka, G. Toda and T. Tanaka, editors.

Summary and future perspectives

Kenichi Kobayashi
First Department of Internal Medicine, School of Medicine, Kanazawa University, Kanazawa 920, Japan

The main theme of this Third Memorial Forum commemorating Dr Tadao Takahashi was literally "hepatocellular carcinoma update" as shown in the subtitle. Each expert in this field of liver disease has presented the brand-new and suggestive data from epidemiology to prevention of hepatocellular carcinoma (HCC). I would like to briefly describe the summary and future perspectives.

Increasing numbers of patients with HCC have been reported in Japan. In 1995, approximately 30,000 people died of primary liver cancer, most of whom had HCC. Liver cancer becomes the third leading cause of cancer death among males and the fourth among females in Japan. However, a rapid decrease might be theoretically possible around the year 2005, because the prevention of HBV and HCV infection has been established in Japan.

It remains controversial whether HCC might be multicentric or not. Multicentric development was shown by detailed pathological investigation and molecular biological techniques. These multicentric characteristics of HCC are clinically a big problem when considering treatment of HCC.

Recent studies support the hypothesis that accumulation of genetic changes underlies the cancer development, and multistep process is well illustrated by colorectal cancer. The relationship between the number of genetic changes and the development of HCC was shown using a new molecular biological technique. Thus, multistep process could be hypothesized also in hepatocarcinogenesis. Based on much more definite evidence, hepatocarcinogenesis must be elucidated in the near future.

The positive ratio of HCV Ab is almost the same between Japan and the USA, compared to the substantial difference of HBsAg-positive rate. The incidence of HCV-related HCC in Japan is much higher than that in the USA. The involvement of HBV DNA in the development of HCV-positive and HBsAg-negative HCCs has been a matter of debate. In order to solve this problem, some researchers have to investigate the actual prevalence of HBV DNA in HBsAg-negative HCCs of the same material by PCR method and Southern blotting, independently.

Address for correspondence: Professor Kenichi Kobayashi MD, First Department of Internal Medicine, School of Medicine, Kanazawa University, Takara-Machi 13-1, Kanazawa 920, Japan. Tel.: +81-762-65-2230. Fax: +81-762-34-4250.

It becomes a daily necessity that the occurrence of HCC-suspected lesions should be examined in the patients of HBV- or HCV-positive chronic liver diseases, regularly and periodically, using mainly abdominal ultrasonography and AFP measurements, especially in Japan. The spread of these screening methods has resulted in the high rate of detection of small HCCs.

In parallel with the progress of diagnosis of HCC, its treatment has also made a rapid progress. Many methodologies have been devised. Surgical treatment, percutaneous ethanol injection and transcatheter arterial embolization are the three major procedures. Various devices have been made for these three methodologies, for example, acetic acid or hot water, instead of ethanol, has been used. Recently, a new radiation therapy using proton beam has been presented and good results have been shown in advanced HCC.

The most favorite method of each institution including the combination treatment should be chosen based on the grade of tumor progression and clinical stage of underlying chronic liver disease.

The very high annual recurrence rate of approximately 20% after the initial successful treatment is very troublesome in either recurrence due to chronological multicentric development or micrometastasis. However, early detection and treatment are essential. Around 10 years survival with good quality of life has to be achieved in all patients with small HCCs detected in a good clinical condition.

Gene therapy for advanced HCC is currently in an experimental stage but results are promising.

Of course, prevention of occurrence of HCC is very important. It has been shown that oral administration of Kampo, the so-called oriental drug, might be effective in decreasing the occurrence of HCC, and that interferon treatment for chronic hepatitis C might also be possible. Retinoic acid has significantly inhibited the recurrence rate of HCC after initial treatment.

Research has been continuing ever since, in order to avoid the occurrence or recurrence of HCC.

I am convinced that all participants should be encouraged to study and to solve many problems in HCC. Finally, I would like to express my sincere gratitude to the organizing committee members of this Memorial Forum.

Index of authors

Keyword index